PENGUIN BOOKS

The Energy Fix

The Energy Fix

Five Steps to Feeling Less Tired

Karina Antram

PENGUIN BOOKS

PENGUIN BOOKS

UK | USA | Canada | Ireland | Australia
India | New Zealand | South Africa

Penguin Books is part of the Penguin Random House group of companies
whose addresses can be found at global.penguinrandomhouse.com

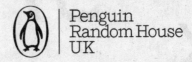

First published as *Fix Your Fatigue* by Penguin Michael Joseph 2023
Published in Penguin Books 2024
001

Printed and bound in Great Britain by Clays Ltd, Elcograf S.p.A.

The authorized representative in the EEA is Penguin Random House Ireland,
Morrison Chambers, 32 Nassau Street, Dublin D02 YH68

A CIP catalogue record for this book is available from the British Library

ISBN: 978-1-405-95470-9

www.greenpenguin.co.uk

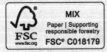

Penguin Random House is committed to a
sustainable future for our business, our readers
and our planet. This book is made from Forest
Stewardship Council® certified paper.

To William, the world is your oyster.

To El, always on my mind, forever in my heart.

Contents

Part 1: LISTENING TO YOUR BODY

Part 2: FIVE STEPS TO FEELING LESS TIRED

Introduction

It's not normal to feel tired all day, every day.

This might surprise you. Everyone's tired, aren't they? Perhaps you think that tiredness is the trade-off for holding down a successful job, having a family, hobbies and an active social life. Well, I want you to realize that it's not, and that life doesn't have to be this way.

Your tiredness might be mild, or it might have become debilitating. It could be a recent experience or a long-standing issue. Perhaps it started with a dip in your performance at work, or maybe you dropped some balls in your personal life, maybe everything slowly got harder and you're not sure when. You might worry that you have lost your edge, or you feel more irritable or emotional than normal. You might even have reached burnout already and lack the energy to do anything at all. On top of that, you're probably masking your symptoms from your family, friends and co-workers, which in itself is exhausting. Perhaps you're even in denial about how tired you feel. You might have tried countless solutions, or you might have tried nothing at all. Why? Because you're too tired.

One thing I do know is that if you've picked up this book,

then you must be fed up with the way you're feeling – the sluggishness, the brain fog, the mild tension headaches, the random aches and pains, the weakness and the gut problems. Because these are just a few of the many symptoms that often accompany ongoing fatigue.

Tiredness, whether mild or debilitating, is your body trying to tell you something. It's saying that whatever you're doing to keep it operating each day isn't working. Something is not right, and the symptoms you're feeling are your body's way of screaming to be heard. This book will help you listen to that cry; it will give you the tools to gain control over your energy and teach you how to never feel tired again. This is exactly the book I needed when I first burnt out.

I never used to think about my health. I was a typical student – drinking copious amounts of alcohol, eating pizza at 3 am and generally enjoying a complete disregard for my body. At the time, I felt invincible. Why would I not? I was having fun, not working, and had very little stress in my life. However, the tell-tale signs of fatigue had already started to show. I was making frequent trips to the doctor about stomach pains, lethargy and sluggishness. I had poor-quality sleep and I didn't exercise. In fact, I was pretty unhealthy. Not that I cared much at the time. But after leaving university, when responsibilities like finding a job and moving to London started to creep up on me, I began to realize that my lifestyle wasn't serving me well.

While working in HR for a well-known consultancy, I started finding it hard to sleep. No matter what I did, I just couldn't switch off my whirring mind and I'd wake up feeling uneasy. This quickly turned into full-blown insomnia, and I started to feel rather strange. I remember going to the gym and not being able to lift even 2kg weights, which are as little as a bag of apples. I had to shower in the bath as I couldn't hold the shower head to wash my hair. Then my symptoms quickly became worse. I started to have panic attacks in the morning on my way into the office and I'd have to calm myself down in the bathroom. It was as if the initial small stressors had eventually layered on top of each other like a Victoria sponge cake, catapulting me into full burnout.

The turning point came one day when I arrived at work feeling as though I was having some sort of out-of-body experience – my mind felt completely disconnected from my body. My boss asked me a question, and all I was able to muster in a very slow, strange voice was: 'I . . . don't . . . know . . . the . . . answer . . . to . . . that.' She looked startled, and I knew at that moment that I really wasn't very well. I couldn't even describe what was wrong with me; all I knew was that I felt very odd. It was like I had cotton wool in place of a brain.

I went straight to the occupational psychologist to ask her what might be wrong. She said that I had burnout and told me to go home. I remember feeling a range of emotions – embarrassment, shame and fear – as I didn't know anyone who had been through a similar experience. I distinctly remember feeling most worried about what my boss and team would think and hoping it could all be kept under wraps. It was the first time I'd ever heard the term 'burnout' as, back then, it wasn't something that was openly discussed in the workplace. But I did what she said and went home to rest.

The trouble was, I only allowed myself two weeks to recuperate. On my first day back I felt very wobbly, and members of the team kept commenting on how much weight I'd lost. I just didn't have an appetite at all. I struggled on for a while, but it quickly became apparent that I'd gone back far too early. I wanted to prove I was resilient and still able to perform, but it had the opposite effect. A few months later, I resigned.

It took me two years to recover from burnout, and even after that I still didn't feel like my old self. I continued to have digestive issues and if I overdid it, I would feel exhausted the next day. The doctors scratched their heads and eventually diagnosed me with chronic fatigue syndrome, or CFS. I realized that if I was to have any chance of once again living a fulfilling life, I had to fix my fatigue for good.

Like anything, my tiredness didn't disappear overnight. It was a combination of many tiny changes that over time contributed to my recovery. Yes, there were some major changes, such as leaving my job, studying and retraining, but it was the small daily changes that had the most impact.

I made my meals as nutrient-dense as possible. I made sure I included a daily walk and some yoga. I took supplements and found ways to destress, developing better connections and focusing on activities that gave me joy so that I didn't waste my precious energy. I tackled a lot of the mental habits I had developed that were contributing to my fatigue. This hasn't been easy, and I have had to play the long game, but it has been worth it. I'm not invincible and, obviously, I still get tired from time to time, but I now have a better work–life balance and feel far more energized than I did before.

It took me a long time to work out what had caused my sudden crash in energy, but now, if I reflect back, it was a combination of several factors. For many years I merely existed in my job. I used to wake up feeling stressed and anxious, hop on the Tube for the inhuman commute rammed with other stressed passengers all looking equally as miserable, and would arrive at work with a smile plastered across my face. I was lured by the money and offer of 'success' and yet the reality was that corporate life wasn't for me. Company cultures didn't align with my values and I found it hard to be creative in a noisy, over-stimulating workplace. I kept picking jobs and environments that did not suit my personality type and values and had a negative impact on my health.

On a physical level, my diet wasn't terrible, but it wasn't great either. I thought I was reasonably healthy but, in reality, I was consuming too many refined sugars, too much alcohol and not enough vegetables, fat and protein. In short, my diet was beige and lacking in micronutrients (vitamins and minerals). I'm a huge fan of food, and although I knew that some of the foods I loved didn't love me back, I wasn't prepared to do anything about it.

Work, diet and lifestyle were the major contributors to my fatigue. Yours might be slightly different, but one thing I know now is that the solutions are the same. Because although my situation was different to yours and my symptoms might have varied, one thing you and I have in common is this: my body was asking for something I was not giving it, and so is yours.

Fixing your fatigue might seem overwhelming. How do you make major changes to your life when you just don't have the energy? I know how that feels, which is why I've developed a simple Five Step process to beat tiredness for good. I won't ask you to overhaul your life, cut out major food groups or go on a radical diet. I will simply show you a system of small, incremental changes that will help you prioritize your health.

I not only helped myself to maximize my general wellbeing, but as a registered nutritionist I have now helped countless others to increase their energy using these Five Steps. In this book I want to share these processes with you so you can also learn how to feel less tired.

This is an evidence-based tiredness toolkit. It's about how you could be eating, sleeping, working, thinking and living to fuel yourself through the good times as well as the tougher times. It combines coaching, psychology and behavioural science with nutrition because these are the tools that will allow you to understand why you make certain choices and will help you make the necessary changes to your behaviour to fix your tiredness for good. By picking up this book, you have already made a great start.

Feeling tired all the time isn't part of life. It's the sound of your body telling you something's wrong. It's now time to listen, understand – and do something about it.

Navigating the Book

I know what it's like when you are completely exhausted. When I was at my most fatigued, I napped for 6 hours a day for 7 months and couldn't work. If someone had given me a book to read on energy, I doubt I would have read it, let alone action the strategies and protocol! Sometimes it all just feels too hard and overwhelming.

I have tried to create a book that feels very easy to read even when you are tired. You don't have to read it all at once if you don't have the energy. You have the choice to dip in and out of the sections that are the most relevant or interesting to you.

The book is divided into two key sections. The first section is trying to get you to think about why you are so tired. It gives you an introduction to many of the causes of fatigue and some simple science about the body to understand how energy is made. The second section introduces the Five Step plan of how you can tackle your tiredness head-on and become more energized.

To help you absorb the information quickly and easily, at the end of each chapter:

- There is a short recap section with the key points from the chapter.
- The science is broken down into easy-to-read simple chunks.
- There is an action for you to start and one reflective question.

You could just read all the summaries from each of the chapters as a start if that is all you feel up to, and as you take the steps towards gaining more energy, you can delve deeper into the sections you'd like.

You can journal in the book too, using the allocated spaces to write and reflect. I also encourage you to revisit the book every month to see how your fatigue feels and assess what steps you have managed to take. Ask yourself, 'Is this having the desired effect or are there more things that I can introduce?'

There is an audio version of the book available if that feels easier to digest and an online course to walk you through the information. Absorb the information in a way that feels right for you and your current state.

At the end of the book, there is also a glossary of terms list if there is one that is unfamiliar and a full list of resources: recommendations for supplements, wellness products and useful directories. Do email me if you have any questions: hello@nocohealth.co.uk. Remember, you are not alone here.

What will you learn from this book?

- Why you may be tired and all the contributing factors.
- How to identify the root cause of your low energy.
- Why the functional medicine approach is the way forward.
- What foods, herbs, supplements and lifestyle Interventions increase energy.
- How to take action when you are already very tired.
- Practical strategies, exercises, tools and reflections.
- A Five Step plan to take you from low to high energy.

Part 1

Listening to Your Body

Chapter 1

Why Am I So Tired?
What is fatigue?

> You feel fine, and then, when your body
> can't keep fighting, you don't.

Nicolas Sparks, *A Walk to Remember*

What's the secret to happiness and fulfilment? Perhaps you think it's your relationships or having a fulfilling purpose in life or simply succeeding in being the person you were meant to be. Perhaps it's a combination of all of these.

I believe the secret to happiness is energy. You might read that statement and think it strange but bear with me. Think about the week you've just had. What have been the biggest threats to your happiness? Maybe you felt tired from work or you argued about something with your partner. Perhaps you felt frustrated by the build-up of admin or chores in the home and, as a result, you weren't able to find the time to exercise, see friends, go on that date night or spend quality time with your family or children.

Now, let's think about what might be behind all of this. Take the argument with your partner, for example. How much better would you have communicated if you hadn't been tired and stressed from work? How much more time would you have had to see friends and family if you hadn't put off doing those jobs around the house? How much more fulfilling would your week at work have been if you'd not felt so run down? When we look closely, we can see that everything, from our relationships to our work to our fulfilment as a person, actually comes down to one thing: energy.

Energy is fundamental to our happiness. And managing our energy is crucial for our physical, social and emotional health. If we don't have enough, our relationships, work and physical wellbeing all suffer. And if we don't address low energy, we can end up masking it by forming addictions – to alcohol, caffeine, sugar, gambling or even prescription or illegal drugs – all to boost our flagging levels and cope with daily life.

Has anybody seen my energy?

So, what makes energy just disappear? To understand this, first we need to know what energy is, how it's made and why it can drop to lower than optimal levels. Then we can begin to unravel some of the personal circumstances that might be affecting *your* energy.

In its simplest form, energy is the 'ability to do work'. However, energy is far more complex than that. I like to think of energy as a resource that supports your physical, mental and emotional needs. If you're properly energized, then you have enough fuel to make it through the day without feeling utterly exhausted or drained. In the right circumstances, our bodies do this brilliantly.

Every single cell in your body needs energy to function and to produce this energy, every cell contains tiny batteries called mitochondria. Mitochondria are the power plants of our cells. Oxidation describes the reaction of a substance with

MITOCHONDRIA

Ribosome
Inner membrane
Intermembrane space
Outer membrane

Matrix
mtDNA
ATP Synthase
ATP (Energy)
Granule
Porin

oxygen. During respiration, food is oxidized to produce energy. In cellular respiration, glucose (a sugar from the food we eat) is oxidized by oxygen (from the air we breathe), producing carbon dioxide, water and energy to fuel our bodies. Mitochondria oxidize carbohydrates, fats and amino acids and convert them into super special molecules called adenosine triphosphate or ATP. ATP molecules are responsible for storing and transferring our energy, so they're a bit like the currency of energy in our bodies. And just like money, we can save up our ATP for when we need it. It's when our energy bank gets low in ATP that we start to feel tired and lethargic. This is because we need ATP to function and if we don't eat the right foods or put our body through too much, our ATP levels decline.

The volume of mitochondria varies within the different cells in our bodies. The heart cells, for example, house 42 per cent of our mitochondria; the kidneys 38 per cent. However, in our brain there is only 5 per cent of our mitochondria, which is frightening really as the brain uses up most of our energy. So, what is the point of this? The point is that we cannot afford to lose any of the mitochondria in our brains. If we do, we will notice a real difference in our brain energy. So many of us struggle with brain fog and our cognition, but what if it is a mitochondrial issue? The question then becomes how do we maintain our brain energy and not lose any precious brain mitochondria?

MAMMALIAN TISSUE MITOCHONDRIAL DENSITY

Tissue	Mitochondrial volume density (% cell volume)	Mitochondrial memb. surface area (m2)/ cm3 of tissue
Heart	42	34
Kidney	38	22
Liver	27	11
Skeletal Muscle	8	12
Lung	6	2
Brain	**5**	**5**

Of course, our energy naturally ebbs and flows like undulating waves in the sea. It depends on many factors, such as how much mental energy you've exerted throughout the day, what you've eaten and how much you've moved. Energy can shift due to emotional or psychological stressors, such as work, illness, grief or trauma, and at different times of the year, with your hormone cycles or along with your work patterns.

But if something goes wrong making our mitochondria – either a lack of vital nutrients in our diet or substances like toxins that block the mitochondria – they can start to dysfunction more permanently. Toxins mostly lead to an increase in oxidative stress, which impairs electron transfer or damages the external structure, leading to a leakage of oxidants. This leakage can then damage other organelles, leading to additional cellular impairment in function. This can cause either a short-term (acute) dip in energy or a longer-term (chronic) type of fatigue, which might be diagnosed as burnout, chronic fatigue syndrome (CFS) or a post-viral fatigue syndrome like Long Covid. The good news is that, because our mitochondria respond to what we do, we can control how they recover, enabling them to create and sustain a continual flow of energy. In the second half of this book, we're going to learn Five Steps that will do just that. But first, it's important to know how to spot the signs of an energy imbalance and try to work out what's causing it.

Spotting energy imbalance

In 2014, Raheem Sterling, by that time already an established England and Liverpool player, was criticized by fans and the media after he asked to opt out of playing in a Euro 2016 qualifier. The reason he gave was that he was too tired. In 2021, Simone Biles, the exceptional US gymnast, withdrew from a number of finals in the Tokyo Olympics, citing her mental wellbeing as the reason. In the same year, tennis player Emma Raducanu was in the last sixteen at Wimbledon and playing brilliantly when she suddenly withdrew from the match for health reasons. Naomi Osaka also withdrew from the French Open in 2021, announcing that she no longer felt happy even when she won a tournament.

All of these professional athletes received a lot of flak at the time, with professional commentators saying they weren't resilient enough. But in all cases, their decision to step back turned out to be the right one for them to protect their energy and wellbeing. According to experts, the number of hours Sterling had played over the two preceding seasons, plus the pressure he felt about his talent at the time, could have created a psychological energy deficit and led to burnout. Yet he anticipated the early signs and, to avoid injury or potentially ending his career, he took himself out of the game and rested. In 2022, he played for England in the World Cup and was a key member of the team.

British professional tennis player Emma Raducanu came

back stronger after taking time out to prioritize her health and competed in the US Open that same year – a tournament she ended up winning. And Simone Biles went on to compete in the Olympic beam final, winning a bronze medal and equalling the record for most medals won by a female gymnast.

All these athletes knew when to quit, change direction or take some much-needed time out *before* they reached burnout. In the same way, the key to maintaining your energy is to spot the warning signs before your energy dips. But how do you know the difference between a temporary lack of energy and a fatigue-related ailment?

If you experience any of the following signs, you might be experiencing the beginning of energy imbalance:

- regularly feeling 'not yourself'
- disturbed sleep
- needing more sleep than normal or napping during the day
- struggling to exercise or experiencing slow recovery from exercise
- feeling weak, dizzy or having headaches
- being more forgetful, not thinking clearly or having 'brain fog'
- feeling more emotional than normal
- moodiness or feeling more irritable than normal
- not feeling as resilient or feeling unable to handle stress

If not caught early, these symptoms of a temporary lack of energy can soon turn into burnout or even a chronic fatigue disorder. Recognizing when you are struggling and taking time out to rest is vital if you don't want to create long-term fatigue.

Spotting burnout

It's easy to see why top athletes get to the point of near-burnout. But what about the rest of us? The fact is that busy jobs, stressful commutes, family pressures and poor lifestyle choices will all have the same effect on our mitochondrial function. The trick is to take time out to focus on yourself before you get to a state of chronic fatigue.

The definition of burnout is the 'prolonged response to chronic interpersonal stressors on the job'. According to the science, there are three key indicators of burnout:

- emotional exhaustion, depletion and loss of energy
- detachment from work
- reduced personal achievement and productivity

If you start to notice that you're doing some or all of the following things, it could be that you are burning out and need to take action:

- emotionally distancing yourself from work, the people in the workplace and feeling increased stress on the job
- experiencing physical symptoms, such as headaches or stomach/digestive-related issues
- experiencing emotional symptoms, such as changes in mood, feeling more tired, an inability to cope with day-to-day life and struggling to control key emotions, such as anger, fear and sadness
- noticing performance changes, like not feeling on your A game or being less creative
- feeling low in confidence or experiencing self-doubt or low motivation

Burnout has similar characteristics to depression and the two can overlap. Likewise, the loss of energy can affect the way we feel, think and act. The problem is that when you are in a de-energized state, people can incorrectly assume that you have depression, when really the issue is poor nutrition and exercise, overworking or not giving enough time to the things you love.

TOP TIP

Make sure you regularly carve out time to check in with yourself and your energy levels. How energized are you feeling right now? How does that compare to last week or last month?

....
....
....
....
....
....

When fatigue becomes chronic

Sometimes, the fatigue we experience in burnout lasts a lot longer. This is known as chronic fatigue, and it can have many causes, but typically it results from:

- a physical illness, such as a virus or, rarely, cancer
- psychological (e.g. depression/anxiety), social (e.g. family stress) or physiological factors (e.g. old age)
- occupational illness (e.g. workplace stress)

Your tiredness might manifest itself in different ways. You might be:

- biochemically tired – when your immune system goes into battle fighting viruses
- physically tired – such as overtraining in the gym
- emotionally tired – if something stressful or sad has happened
- physiologically tired – due to lack of sleep
- cognitively tired – if you have spent too much time making decisions or at a computer
- cellularly tired – if your cells haven't got the right nutrients to create ATP, causing fatigue

Or a combination of some or all of these.

If your energy problems have been going on for more than 6 months, you could have chronic fatigue syndrome or CFS. For many years CFS wasn't recognized as a genuine illness, yet in recent years research has shown that it does indeed exist and can impact our lives greatly without treatment and life-style changes. Because there isn't one test that confirms the diagnosis, symptoms of CFS often leave doctors scratching their heads and it's often misdiagnosed as depression, anxiety or other conditions.

CFS is normally confirmed if fatigue that does not improve with rest has occurred for more than 6 months and there are other symptoms such as:

- impaired memory or concentration
- sore throat
- tender lymph nodes
- muscle pain
- multi-joint pain
- new headaches
- unrefreshing sleep
- post-exercise fatigue

In my worst periods of CFS, I struggled to get out of bed and would be extremely fatigued all day. I found the smallest of tasks difficult, such as brushing my hair, and at times I struggled to eat as I had no appetite. But perhaps the most difficult thing about CFS was the lack of concrete answers. Each time I saw the doctors they requested blood to be taken but each time there didn't appear to be anything wrong with me. What I really needed was a proper protocol to follow, with some dietary and lifestyle guidance and reassurance that I could improve my symptoms through these mechanisms alone.

How tired are you?

One of the reasons we accept tiredness for so long is because it can creep up on us. That's why spotting the signs of burnout or encroaching chronic fatigue is so important. So right now, how tired are you? Take a look at the scale opposite and mark on it where you would put your energy levels at this moment.

This will involve stopping what you are doing and really listening to your body, so don't rush your answer. Writing down and then seeing how tired you are on the page in front of you will help you make the connection. You'll be able to see that there is a path to improvement as you can see the stages above you.

HOW TIRED ARE YOU?

5	4	3	2	1
Total Fatigue & Exhaustion – Nothing Left	Very Fatigued	Moderately Fatigued	A Little Fatigued	Not Fatigued At All

(Micklewright et al., 2017)

Whatever you answer, remember this: your tiredness can improve. You will not be at that level forever. And once you understand your energy issues, everything starts to change. You'll think more clearly, feel happier and calmer, achieve more during the day, have a better impact on other people and even feel more confident and self-assured. The list is endless. Once you make the decision to prioritize creating and maintaining energy, you will feel like a different person. In fact, I'd like to bet that if you implement even some of the changes in this book and revisit this scale in a month, your score will be lower.

But before we start to explore those changes, we need to find out what's making YOU tired. And to do this we need to discover what's using up your energy.

TTDR (TOO TIRED DIDN'T READ)

If you are too tired to read the full chapter, here is a brief recap of what you have missed:

- Energy is vital for your happiness and at the centre of your energy is YOU.
- Symptoms of fatigue go beyond tiredness. They can include digestive issues, brain fog, muscle pain and headaches, so don't ignore these.
- You might not realize how tired you are because you are masking it from those around you. Measure yourself honestly on the tiredness scale.
- If you are heading for burnout you might need to quit something, change direction or take time out. Think of ways you could do this NOW.

SCIENCE

Most of our energy is created by mitochondria, tiny organelles that live in our cells. They create ATP, which is the currency of energy in our bodies. ATP can be 'saved' for when we need it, just like money, but only if we pace ourselves.

ONE ACTION

Write a list of the symptoms you experience regularly and when they are at their worst.

ONE QUESTION

When did your fatigue really start? Was there a triggering event or situation?

Chapter 2

Who Stole My Energy?
Energy leaks and how to spot them

The energy of the mind is the essence of life.

Aristotle

COMMON FACTORS THAT IMPACT ENERGY

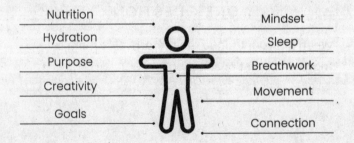

Nutrition | Mindset
Hydration | Sleep
Purpose | Breathwork
Creativity | Movement
Goals | Connection

A phrase I often hear when I see clients at my clinic is: 'Tell me why I'm tired!' They, like everyone who experiences chronic fatigue, just want to know why they have so little energy. But while I wish I could give them a straight answer there and then, the reality is that knowing why you're so tired isn't usually that simple. In fact, often there is no single answer to this question at all, which is why many of my clients have already been on a long and fruitless journey with their doctor. Blood tests have come back normal, scans show nothing, and yet they are still tired. So where has their energy gone?

Of course, our body uses energy just to stay alive. Here are some of the processes that use up our energy before we even do anything:

- blood circulation
- cell growth
- respiration
- neurological reactions
- digestion and absorption

Then there are 'events' that use energy, such as:

- injury or trauma
- our emotions
- illness
- exercise

But on top of this are the many factors that contribute to energy loss without giving us any gains. I call these our energy 'leaks'. How these factors impact you will differ from person to person due to genetics and your own individual biochemistry, and it's this individuality that means the cause of your fatigue is probably unique to you.

Someone with quite obvious energy 'leaks' was Laura. She was in her early fifties when she came to see me and she was suffering from poor sleep, anxiety and depression. She was grieving the loss of her parent and had been diagnosed with Long Covid. She was doing everything right when it came to diet and exercise and yet she couldn't shift her debilitating fatigue, weakness and lethargy. As a result, she was feeling very demotivated.

I quickly realized that as Laura was eating a nutritionally dense diet already, something else was draining her energy. Her body was making ATP, but as fast as she could make it, she was losing it. We didn't need to delve too deep to discover that Laura was processing a lot of grief and this was causing her emotional fatigue. As she was experiencing poor sleep, she was physiologically tired and her body wasn't getting the rest and recovery she desperately needed.

As Laura was very tired we started by making small changes. I suggested that we focus on improving her sleep and reducing her mental fatigue, so I recommended she take a specifically formulated sleep supplement containing Montmorency cherry, a natural source of melatonin (the sleep hormone) and magnesium. I suggested she attend bereavement counselling to help her to process her grief. Once Laura was feeling better, we decided to introduce an activity to increase her mental energy and take her mind off things, so she joined a cookery class. As a result, she discovered a new community of like-minded people.

For Laura, grief and poor sleep were causing her energy to 'leak', gradually causing an energy deficit. It's these leaks that are often the clue to the cause of our fatigue.

What are your leaks?

Envisage a bowl with a hole in it. Even if the hole is very tiny, any water put in that bowl will gradually seep out. It's the same with our energy. Any 'holes' we have in our life – aspects of our current situation that use up a lot of our energy – will cause energy leaks. Once sealed, the bowl can remain full, but without the sealant, the leaks will reappear.

Some energy leaks are universal and will apply to most of us. These are things like stress, work, family, juggling multiple responsibilities and financial pressures. But there are probably some others you haven't previously considered, such as:

- smoking
- social media
- not planning your days and wasting your time on things that don't bring you joy
- lack of sunlight
- sitting all day at a computer or watching TV

To understand why *you* in particular are experiencing fatigue, we need to look into all the possible energy leaks that could be affecting you. We need to remember that these forces are bi-directional: they impact both the mind and the body, like a two-way street. They can be categorized into mental, physical, emotional and self-fulfilment factors, but some energy leaks – such as stress – will cover all four.

Mental

Stress

If I were to ask you to describe a stressful experience, you'd probably tell me about a major life quake such as being made redundant, going through a divorce or losing a loved one. What you might not think about are the smaller, more insidious sources of stress that can build up without us realizing. In *When the Body Says No*, Gabor Maté explains that the three factors that are most likely to lead to stress are in fact uncertainty, lack of information and the loss of control. Here are some examples of ongoing stress that you might not have noticed:

- overworking
- decision fatigue – having too many decisions to make
- illness
- caring responsibilities
- social isolation

Psychological stressors like these affect not only the energy we have but the energy we give off and the energy we expend. In fact, 'micro-stressors' built up over a long duration can have a catastrophic effect on our minds and bodies – they make us sick, cause us to crave bad food and can create permanent digestive problems, like IBS. When you understand what stress does to our systems, this makes sense. As Maté explains, stress disproportionately affects the endocrine system (hormones), the immune system and the digestive system.

Whether stress is acute with a rapid onset (usually due to a triggering event) or chronic – that is, it has built up over a long period of time – it is difficult to escape. The modern lifestyle most of us lead – long working hours, commuting, balancing work with family, 24/7 accountability, the new blend of work life and home life and constant technology – can be a serious energy leak.

Anxiety/depression

Did you know that the brain represents just 2 per cent of your body's weight yet uses 20 per cent of your energy? (Hyder et al., 2013). And that's just your resting brain. If the brain performs a task, such as taking an exam, its energy consumption increases by 5 per cent. Now imagine you are doing all of that *and* you are battling the negative or catastrophic thoughts that come with anxiety or depression. Poor mental health uses a huge amount of energy and is one of the biggest energy leaks, which is why people suffering from depression often experience physical exhaustion.

Mindset

However, you don't have to be clinically depressed for your brain to become an energy leak. In the same way as depression can cause tiredness, a pattern of negative thinking and worrying can drain the brain's energy. Pessimism can even reduce the effectiveness of your immune system (Lee et al., 2022), making you more susceptible to illness and less able to recover.

Discover how to manage negative thoughts and conserve brain energy on pages 202 and 204.

Physical

Nutrition

If we don't consume the right fats, carbohydrates, protein sources and micronutrients (vitamins and minerals) or if we eat too much sugar, additives, unhealthy trans fats and alcohol, the body will simply not function to the best of its ability. It is estimated 60 per cent of the UK/US diet is processed (Martínez et al., 2016; Rauber et al., 2019) and most of the food the world consumes isn't even really food. Even if you're not over-eating, what you do and do not eat could be seriously affecting your health and your energy levels.

Breathing

The way you breathe not only affects how you feel but has a direct effect on your nervous system. When life's stressors take hold, it's easy to get into a habit of breathing from your chest rather than your stomach or even to hold your breath for periods of time. Habitual over-breathing or taking shallow breaths can increase anxiety and affect the way you respond to stress because it reduces the amount of oxygen that can get into your cells. It increases your heart rate and raises your blood pressure. All this can have a catastrophic effect on your energy levels. We'll look at some simple breathing techniques in Step 5 (see page 213).

Sleep

Sleep is so crucial for cellular repair that humans cannot survive for more than two weeks without it. Sleep can be classified into REM and non-REM sleep and is regulated by melatonin and the sleep/wake cycles known as circadian rhythms. A lack of sleep can cause a whole host of symptoms and chronic insomnia can become debilitating. Even if you are regularly getting a little less than you need, lack of sleep can become an energy leak.

Gut health

An imbalance of bad and good bacteria in the gut (dysbiosis) doesn't just cause digestive issues. It can heavily impact energy, making you feel sluggish and causing brain fog and general malaise. In fact, many conditions are now thought to start in the gut, so becoming knowledgeable about how to nourish and heal your gut is key in supporting many energy-related conditions. The great thing is that the gut microbiome (see page 239) is adaptable – it can change and it can get better. This is known as gastro plasticity. We'll learn more about how to improve gut health in Step 2 (see page 144).

Movement

We know that exercise is good for us, but when it comes to energy production it can be a double-edged sword. Daily movement not only uses energy but creates it, so moving your body is the easiest, quickest way of picking yourself up when you're feeling tired. However, the wrong type of movement at the wrong time or overdoing it with excessive exercise can have a negative effect on your body. In other words, regular exercise in moderation creates 'good' stress, but if you're already stressed, exhausted or unwell, pushing yourself to do that HIIT workout will only make you worse. In fact, it's been proven that excessive exercise isn't necessary to improve your health. A 2019 study of all women found that walking 4,400 steps a day reduced mortality rates, but the reduction in risk maxed out at 7,500 steps, so there's simply no need to push yourself to do the recommended 10,000 steps (Lee et al., 2019). Knowing this and being strategic about how and when to exercise – not forcing yourself to exercise at the wrong times – will help you conserve your energy and avoid exercise becoming an energy leak.

Hydration

A lack of fluid (and this doesn't include fizzy or caffeinated drinks and alcohol) can become a major energy leak as it causes your cells to become dehydrated and reduce blood flow to the brain. Again, how much you need to drink will depend on a number of factors, such as climate, how much you sweat, whether you are exercising or even if you are breastfeeding. As a guideline, we should be aiming to consume 1.5–2 litres of fluid every day.

Age

Fatigue can occur at any age due to the different milestones of life, but one thing we all have in common is that our energy naturally wanes as we age. One of the causes of this is micronutrient deficiencies – in other words, a lack of essential vitamins and minerals – due to a decrease in absorption as we get older. Obviously, ageing is an energy leak we can't do much about but supporting micronutrient status with supplements is one way of combating this natural reduction in energy.

Gender

Unfortunately, women often struggle with low energy more than men because of the milestones in their reproductive life. Starting periods and subsequent blood loss, pregnancy, childbirth, postnatal recovery, perimenopause and menopause can all cause hormonal dysregulation, which can severely impact energy levels. But fatigue due to imbalanced hormones can occur in both sexes if the (oestrogen, testosterone and progesterone) levels aren't quite right.

Breastfeeding

Since having had my babies, I now know what it takes to feed a little one. The energy struggle is real! One of the ways I'm able to keep my energy up is to take a specific breastfeeding formulation so that my micronutrient status doesn't deplete. It's thought that it takes around a year for a woman's iron levels to go back to normal after childbirth, so taking a specific multivitamin alongside a good-quality absorbable iron supplement is a big help during this stage, though it is worth getting your iron levels tested first. But again, all women have different pregnancies, labours and requirements, so the type of support you need will vary.

Weight and eating patterns

Society is quick to judge those who are obese, but the truth is that any weight-related disorder can lead to micronutrient deficiencies and therefore become an energy leak. Under-eating is just as bad for your health as overeating, so it's important to find the weight that suits you and your body type. This can be difficult to achieve but undereating or overeating can be highly inflammatory for the body so neither end of the spectrum is beneficial.

Knowing how much to eat and when to eat it is hard, which is why we'll look in detail at emotional vs intuitive eating in Step 1 (see page 137). Yet again, there isn't a one-size-fits-all approach, which is why I recommend ditching the scales (and the BMI calculator).

Deficiencies and toxins

Typically, when your body starts to show symptoms it's either because of low micronutrient status, i.e. deficiencies in vitamins and minerals, or a high level of toxins. We live in a toxic world and unfortunately we can't escape exposure to many of the toxins that come from pollution, cleaning products, toiletries, perfumes, medicines, paint, candles made from paraffin wax and many other products. Toxins block the production of energy in the mitochondria, so can quite easily become an energy leak.

Seasonality

You won't meet many people who say they have more energy in the winter than in the summer. Most of us tend to feel the need to hibernate in the colder months, and some of us would even say we suffer from SAD (seasonal affective disorder). This is because in winter the body is really asking us to conserve our energy. When we don't move as much or get adequate vitamin D, we can feel lethargic and unmotivated, and simply the time of year can become an energy leak.

TOP TIP ✏️

If you have noticeably less energy in the winter, consider taking a vitamin D supplement between October and April and take a short walk outdoors first thing in the morning.

Emotional

Emotions

If you're one of those people who feels emotions more deeply than others, whether that's sadness, grief, trauma, excitement or simply the impact of events in the news, you might be what Elaine Aron calls a 'highly sensitive person (HSP)' (Aron, 1996). If your lack of control over your emotions causes you to ruminate, overthink or catastrophize, you can quickly start to feel fatigued. Understanding yourself and who you are, together with emotional thought management, can help you to process these types of deeper emotions and stop them being an energy leak.

Even if you're not an HSP, emotional suppression can lead to fatigue and even ill health. Learning to cultivate more positive emotions and allowing yourself to feel the harder emotions can be beneficial for your energy.

If you're a Highly Sensitive Person, find out more about how to manage yourself on page 215.

Connection

According to theories in positive psychology, connection is the key to happiness. For many of us, lockdown and social distancing have reduced the strength of our connections and for those of us who gain energy from others, this will have negatively impacted our energy levels. Those with an E (extrovert) personality type on the Myers-Briggs scale may have struggled more with this loss of connection, which can subsequently affect our internal motivation and become an energy leak. While the world has never been more connected through social media, there has been an increase in loneliness. Being lonely or having fewer social connections can even change our brains, with grey matter being greater and default networks more tightly wired together (Spreng et al., 2020).

Introverts versus extroverts

We all gain and lose energy in different ways. Being an introvert, I can lose my energy very quickly by being around people for too long. I'm the type of person who, if you see me for a few hours, I can be on form, but if I'm talking to people for too long I get easily drained and need to leave. Extroverts like my partner don't have this predicament and feel energized by being around lots of people most of the time but conversely feel lower in energy when alone. Not understanding the type of character you are and managing your energy accordingly can become an energy leak.

Self-fulfilment

Purpose

Whether you are ambitious and driven or not, everyone needs to have a purpose. If you don't have a 'why', a reason to get up in the morning and crack on successfully with your day, it can have a serious impact on your energy. For me, my purpose is to support and help people with their health and wellbeing so that they have the energy to live their lives to the fullest. It's also to make sure I'm the best mother to my family, so that they have a happy and successful life. Purpose is about having something to focus on that is greater than yourself – the self-actualization point on any coaching model.

Goals

As well as having a purpose, my father taught me the art of having a BHAG – a Big, Hairy, Audacious Goal. This means having one goal that really excites you but feels completely out of reach. My BHAG (which I have to say still feels out of reach!) has always been to buy my own waterside bolthole by a beach in Europe, so I can escape the winters in the UK (I'm not a fan of the cold). I don't know if I will ever achieve it, but it's something to aim for and it's good to dream. Scientists Edwin Locke and Gary Latham conducted a study that showed that setting a BHAG improved performance more than having a general 'do your best' mentality. They found that it was the most difficult goals that stimulated the highest levels of effort and performance. Conversely, not having something to work towards can be a drain on energy, so it's important to have exciting goals you can aim for daily. Dopamine, our reward neurotransmitter, increases when we set a goal and when we are close to achieving it. The brain likes challenging goals. The dopamine spike is increased when the goal is harder to attain (Mohebi et al., 2019).

Creativity

Sometimes a lack of fun or the inability to be creative can be a sap on your energy. Everyone expresses creativity differently, but not being able to express it at all can add to stress and contribute to feelings of unhappiness. Similarly, boredom is a major energy leak, as the same receptors in the brain that are responsible for enjoying ourselves will induce tiredness if left unstimulated. Researchers have found that when we want to fall asleep, say in a boring lecture or meeting, it's because the nucleus accumbens, a key region in the brain responsible for our behaviours involved in pleasure and motivation, can also elicit sleep (Oishi et al., 2017).

This tells us that our environment can have a profound impact on our energy levels. Have you ever noticed that when you are in the right environment that your energy levels are really high, but when you are listening to or doing something that you don't enjoy, you feel sleepy? This is why choosing the right workplace is so important for productivity and performance.

Now, you may think that dialling up your activity to include creativity-laden activities is the answer, but sometimes just having more time and space to think is best according to Einstein, who said, 'Creativity is the residue of time wasted.' It is the balance between being in a creatively stimulating environment that you find intrinsically motivating and having enough time and space away to spark the creativity in the first place. According to Austin Kleon, 'Creative people need time to just sit around and do nothing.' So if you are a highly creative person, make sure you factor time in each day to do just that!

Personality type

Genetics account for 8 per cent of the difference in people's tiredness and low energy (Deary et al., 2018). If your mother or father has always struggled with their energy, there's a small chance that you could have a genetic susceptibility towards fatigue. According to other studies, there are personality traits that make an individual more susceptible to fatigue or burnout. These characteristics are typically:

- hard-working
- perfectionist
- obsessive-compulsive
- overactive

(Greenberg, 2002)

If any of these sound like you, then your personality type and the way you typically interact with others could be an energy leak. The following personality types can experience low energy. See if any of them resonate with you.

The supporter

You keep giving to others but forget to top up your own energy reserves, resulting in energy leaks.

The mood depleter

You focus on past events, ruminating on what you could have done differently or failed at. As a result, you struggle to root yourself in the present day.

The futuristic

You focus too much on the future and don't live fully in the present.

The overthinker

You are always in fight or flight mode, which uses up a lot of energy. You often give thoughts far too much time and attention, creating fear or anxiety about what is to come.

The captive

If your family or friends are going through a tough time, you have a tendency to absorb these emotions. This can eat away at energy.

Your unique chronotype

Sometimes, traditional medicine assumes that all bodies are the same, and I believe this is why doctors often fail to discover why someone is chronically tired. The reality is we each have lots of unique inner clocks that control our energy, mood and sleep (Turek and Jiang, 2017). In fact, we have clocks in every organ of our body. We each have a specific chronotype that is decided by the length of a particular gene that, in turn, is dependent on genetic, environmental and age-related factors. Knowing your chronotype will ensure that you develop an innate understanding of when to use and conserve your energy throughout the day at the right times.

Which chronotype you are will dictate what time of the day you prefer to exercise, eat and sleep. It explains why some people are night owls and others are more energized in the morning and why some people don't feel like eating breakfast (Maukonen et al., 2016). According to the research, those with an evening chronotype are said to consume less whole grains, rye, potatoes, vegetables and roots but consume more wine and chocolate (Kanerva et al., 2012). Your chronotype can affect all aspects of your lifestyle, not just your sleep.

Most importantly, failing to understand your chronotype can have a serious impact on your energy levels. If you are constantly fighting against your chronotype – for example, getting up early when you are naturally an evening type – you may find yourself out of tune with your body. This can result in lower energy levels. If you find the right schedule for your sleep, eating and activity you will be more aligned with your inner body clock, which may have a positive impact on your energy levels. Even fitting your activities or work around your chronotype could be beneficial.

Our unique chronobiology determines what is right for us. This is why we shouldn't base all our decisions on scientific research or simply follow the latest fad diet. Instead, we need to tap into what our bodies need and then eat, move and sleep at the right times for us.

Feeling out of sorts? Our internal clocks may be out of sync, known as 'clock dysfunction'. We have clocks for light, food and exercise, but most of us are out of kilter, caused by electric light and screen time. If we ignore our natural bedtimes, wake up late, skip meals or don't exercise regularly, this creates 'clock dysfunction'.

This can affect energy, metabolism and mood. Being permanently out of whack can increase insomnia, depression and diabetes.

To reset your clocks Professor Russell Foster, expert in circadian neuroscience at Oxford University, suggests:

- Never go to sleep on an argument – the stress hormones shorten sleep.
- Write down all your thoughts before bed to reduce the stress hormones impacting your sleep.
- Thirty minutes of sunlight (without sunglasses) before 9 am resets your clock at the beginning of the day. The sunlight triggers a neural circuit that controls the timing of the hormones cortisol, also known as glucocorticoid, and melatonin, which

affect sleep. A morning walk also calms you, known as 'optic flow'. Interestingly, this circuit quietens when you walk past moving objects, reducing stress.

- Thirty minutes of natural light before sunset resets your clock for the evening to ensure we get enough melatonin to encourage sleep.
- Stick to regular bedtimes to allow your body to find its natural rest mode setting in the evenings.
- Leave a 14-hour window before eating to give your microbiome a rest, so stop eating dinner at 7 pm and have breakfast at 9 am.

If you are in need of a reset, try these tips for a month and see if it makes a difference to how you feel.

Finding the source of your energy leaks is vital when beginning to investigate your fatigue. And as you can see, many factors affect our energy, not just diet and sleep. You might recognize some of the leaks in this chapter, or there might be others that are unique to you. Looking at your whole lifestyle is crucial when trying to determine what's wrong, as only when we understand our unique set of mental, physical, emotional and self-fulfilment circumstances can we begin to find out why we're tired.

TTDR (TOO TIRED DIDN'T READ)

- Energy is used for all our bodily processes, from digestion to brain function.
- Our energy 'leaks' are unique to us, but there are some common culprits we can look out for, such as stress.
- Physical energy leaks like dehydration, over-exercising or eating too little could be contributing to your fatigue.
- Even our personality type can affect how we spend and conserve our energy and whether we are at greater risk of burnout.
- Our unique inner body clock is called our chronotype and it affects how and when we eat, sleep and move. Ignoring your chronotype and forcing yourself to sleep, eat or exercise at the wrong time of day could be causing a reduction in energy.

SCIENCE

We each have a specific chronotype that is decided by the length of a particular gene that, in turn, is dependent on genetic, environmental and age-related factors. Knowing your chronotype will ensure that you develop an innate understanding of when to use and conserve your energy throughout the day at the right times.

ONE ACTION

Keep a note for a week that captures when you have the most energy. Is it in the morning, the middle of the day or the evening? What do you notice?

ONE QUESTION

Which energy 'leaks' in this chapter did you recognize?

Chapter 3

How Can I Mend My Broken Mitochondria?
The science of energy

It's mitochondria not hypochondria.

Dr Sarah Myhill

In the last chapter we turned detective to look at which energy leaks might be contributing to your fatigue. Whichever of these leaks resonated with you, they have one thing in common: they affect how we make and use energy. Understanding how our bodies do this will help us discover a little more about why you're tired – and how to fix it. To do this, we need to get back to the mitochondria.

Samira came to see me presenting with exhaustion. The reasons were not particularly clear even as I was going through her case. She had been very tired for many years. She seemingly ate quite a good, balanced, nutrient-dense diet, although there was a marked difference in volume on some days versus others and she did consume some processed meals on the days she felt tired. She did some form of movement most days, mostly low-impact yoga and walking. She worked in marketing and had a good, stable home life. She recently had some blood tests at the GP that came back normal. I was left scratching my head. Everything seemed good, yet she felt terrible.

When we delved into her full case history, something became apparent. She admitted to having an eating disorder for a number of years. While her weight was now stable and she said she had recovered, some years prior she was very undernourished. With that information to hand, it could be that her mitochondria were not in abundance as much as they should be. Anorexia causes oxidative stress, which can create mitochondrial dysfunction. I had to play detective and try something that I thought could provide some relief.

We needed to get more energy into her cells by fuelling the mitos and create an environment where her mitos could thrive. I introduced more healthy fats into her diet, crucial fuel for the mitos, in the form of avocados, coconut flakes, nuts and seeds. We made sure her meals were more consistent every day, rather than some days eating a lot more food than others, to ensure her mitos were getting consistent fuel every day. We removed all of the processed food she was consuming to reduce inflammation and instead replaced it with home-cooked, simple and easy-to-digest meals, such as stews, soups and one-pot, tray-baked dishes with lots of vegetables. I asked her to take D-Ribose, a supplement essential in energy production.

I asked what stressors Samira had in her life as stress can

impair mito function and she mentioned that her job wasn't providing the satisfaction that it once did and she felt her performance was dipping. I suggested that she look at moving horizontally within her company into a new role, moving out of her company into the same role, or retraining and do something entirely different.

For her follow-up she came back delighted. You could see the energy change just by her face. She had fully embraced the new lifestyle and said her eating habits were the most consistent they had been for years. She decided to stay in marketing but become a freelancer to give her greater flexibility, which made a huge difference to her quality of life.

The energy bank

We know from Chapter 1 that energy production in our cells is the job of the mitochondria and that their role is to take the energy from food and turn it into ATP. We referred to ATP as the currency of energy because, like money, we can't really operate without it.

Under normal circumstances our bodies are good at storing ATP, always keeping some in the bank so we have energy when we need it. To do this they use an efficient recycling system so that when we've used some ATP, we can take energy from the nutrients in our food to make more.

Having stored ATP means that when we suddenly have to run for a bus or make a difficult decision, we have enough energy to do so. But ATP doesn't just give us energy, it's also vital for keeping the biological pathways of our body going.

Imagine a system of roads. This system connects places and people together, and without it we couldn't get to where we need to go. The same can be said for the pathways in our body. Take hormones, for example. Our hormones need to travel within the bloodstream. If these hormones don't have enough ATP to take them there, they will break down. When our biological pathways don't flow properly, we're at higher risk of disease or illness. So mitochondria and ATP are vital not only for how well we *feel*, but for how well we actually *are*.

When mitochondria go wrong

So, what about people with chronic fatigue? Well, there's a lot we still don't know about mitochondria but we do know that, to work well, our ATP recycling process needs to happen around every ten seconds. However, for people with fatigue issues ATP is only able to recycle around once a minute (Myhill, 2017). Over time, this means a chronic lack of energy.

We don't exactly know why mitochondria dysfunction in some people and not in others, but research has shown that mitochondria can stop functioning well if they:

- have a poor environment OR
- are pushed too hard – pacing yourself is key!

Let's look at what a poor environment means first. A poor environment for mitochondria could be due to any – or all – of the following:

- processed foods that lack the important nutrients the mitos need
- toxins
- stress

Now, we're not going to talk about calories in this book (you'll see why in Step 1 later on – see page 105), but we should be interested in how our bodies digest, absorb and metabolize certain foods. This is known as the thermic effect of foods, or TEF. In other words, it takes energy to make energy. The interesting thing to know about TEF is that it takes more energy to digest and absorb highly processed foods than nutrient-dense, whole foods. Think about that for a minute – processed foods require more energy from your mitochondria just to get the nutrients into the bloodstream. So, when we eat junk food, not only is it not providing adequate nutrition for our body, but we waste a whole lot of ATP just to digest it. And then those foods are inflammatory to the body. Over time, this can create an energy deficit as the mitos struggle to keep up with production of ATP.

Stress and toxins create a poor environment for our mitochondria (we'll learn more about toxins in Step 2 on page 149). This is because when we're stressed, mitochondria in the adrenal glands produce the stress hormone cortisol. We might

WHERE IS ENERGY USED IN THE BODY?

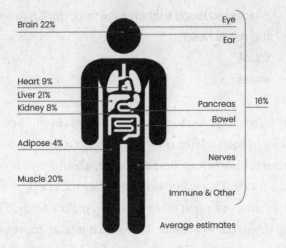

Brain 22%

Eye

Ear

Heart 9%

Liver 21%

Kidney 8%

Pancreas

16%

Bowel

Adipose 4%

Nerves

Muscle 20%

Immune & Other

Average estimates

think of cortisol as bad, but actually it performs a vital function in the body. It stimulates the 'fight or flight' response and tells our cells to produce more energy to deal with whatever is threatening us. It's what would allow us to run away from a wild animal or, in more modern terms, step quickly away from the road if a car is coming.

But what happens when our mitochondria are having to make cortisol *all the time*?

Under constant stress, the mitochondria can become overworked. Scientists are still researching what effect making too much cortisol has on mitochondria, but it's thought that it makes them produce more of the molecules known as Reactive

Oxygen Species, or ROS. ROS is toxic for cells and, over time, it damages the mitochondria so they don't work so well.

So, it's clear that while acute periods of stress aren't necessarily bad for us, ongoing stress (often known as toxic stress) might have serious consequences for our energy production.

Another factor that can damage our mitochondria is pushing them too hard and one way we do this is through excessive exercise. Now, obviously exercise is key to good health and moving our bodies is important in combating fatigue, but over-exercising and over-exertion can be detrimental to our energy levels. A recent study showed that those who did HIIT training strenuously most days developed a severe decline in mito function in addition to blood sugar dysfunction. Whilst studies show short bursts of intense exercise increase the number of mitochondria, those who worked out moderately five times a week compared to those who worked out with HIIT three times a week saw a greater difference in body fat and blood pressure (Flockhart et al., 2021). This is because pushing yourself hard requires a greater use of energy to power up our bodies. When this happens, our mitochondria go into overdrive and they can't recycle ATP as efficiently, so our reserves get low. When they deplete, we don't have enough energy to function, let alone do that 5k run. This is why many people with CFS experience what's known as post-exertional fatigue. Pushing yourself too hard for too long can build up to a chronic lack of energy.

Another factor that can push our mitochondria too hard is illness and infection. If you've had a virus, such as glandular fever (Epstein-Barr), flu or Covid-19, you might experience ongoing tiredness that lasts long after the initial illness. In some cases, this can develop into chronic fatigue and be accompanied by other symptoms, such as brain fog and muscle aches. This is because the body needs a lot of energy in the form of ATP to fight the infection and your ATP levels may have become depleted as a result (Segerstrom, 2007). Add in a lack of appetite, which often accompanies viral illnesses, and your body will struggle to take in the nutrients it needs to produce replacement energy.

As we learnt from our energy leaks, another factor that results in our mitochondria being pushed too hard is under-eating or overeating, so if you are over- or under-eating you could be inadvertently reducing your mitochondria's ability to produce a steady flow of energy. This is especially true in the case of mixing the two – in other words, yo-yo dieting. Inconsistent eating creates dysregulation in how hungry or full we feel. When we starve ourselves only to give in and overeat later because we are so hungry, we disrupt our blood sugar, which makes life hard for our mitochondria.

To understand whether you are doing this, take a look at the hunger diagram opposite. On a normal day, where do you usually fall on this scale before a meal? Do you tend to wait until you are ravenous until you eat something, are you a planner or sometimes do you overestimate how much you need and feel uncomfortable after?

THE HUNGER SCALE

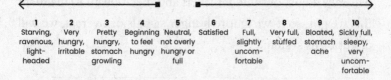

1	2	3	4	5	6	7	8	9	10
Starving, ravenous, light-headed	Very hungry, irritable	Pretty hungry, stomach growling	Beginning to feel hungry	Neutral, not overly hungry or full	Satisfied	Full, slightly uncomfortable	Very full, stuffed	Bloated, stomach ache	Sickly full, very uncomfortable

Being either at 1 or 10 on the scale isn't good for us. Instead, we should be identifying when we get hungry at around 4 and start to prepare food. Likewise, when we're eating we should learn to stop at around 6 so that we avoid overeating and feeling sluggish and lethargic.

Obesity places a particular strain on our mitochondria because it causes inflammation in the body. In a study of 49 pairs of twins in Helsinki in 2021, biopsies were taken of each participant's fat and muscle tissue. When researchers studied the mitochondria, they found that those who were suffering with obesity had reduced mitochondrial function in the fat tissue, meaning their body was struggling to produce enough energy in those cells. The relationship between obesity and mitochondrial function is a two-way street: when mito function is reduced, it can maintain obesity. And just as idling in a car produces toxic exhaust fumes, a low mito engine releases toxins into the body that can lead to a pro-inflammatory state and subsequent obesity-related diseases (Van der Kolk et al., 2021).

The good news is that our bodies have an internal thermostat that is designed to regulate our weight. This set point, or hedonic adaptation, is the range where our weight sits most happily. The reason yo-yo dieting is so bad is because our brains naturally adjust our hunger levels and metabolism to maintain this weight, so if we ignore hunger signals or overeat, we will disrupt this system.

For information on how to practise intuitive eating to maintain your set point weight, turn to page 138.

Our mitochondria hold the key to our energy levels. Creating a good environment where they can thrive and avoiding pushing them too hard are vital if we want to maintain a steady flow of energy.

Hormetic stressors

Another great way to increase the volume of your mitochondria is by 'mitohormesis' which is a mild cellular stress, encouraging mitochondria to generate low levels of ROS which initiates a stress defense mechanism, protecting cells from further damage. Hormetic stressors such as heat stress from saunas or cold stress from ice baths, exercise and fasting can all contribute to better health. (Yoon et al., 2022.)

Exposure to heat such as a sauna session can reduce symptoms of depression and improve mood. A hot bath, which creates something known as heat shock proteins, can also be used. These improve innate immunity, increase the number of immune cells and improve blood sugar control. (Faulkner et al., 2017.)

The opposite hormetic stressor is cold exposure. Using cold therapy creates the biogenesis of new mitochondria. (Chung et al., 2017.) The most effective combination is practicing a breathing exercise in conjunction with cold exposure which decreases the inflammatory response of the body. (Zwaag et al., 2022.) Catecholamines (including dopamine, adrenaline and noradrenaline) increase in ways that can improve your focus, concentration and mood. The quality of stress caused by deliberate cold exposure is most likely to lead to one of 'eustress' – associated with positive health outcomes.

To maximize the benefits of cold therapy, the environment should be uncomfortably cold but such that you can stay in safely. Cold water immersion up to the neck is the most effective way, but a cold shower is the next best thing if you can't brave a full immersion.

However, there are other factors that can harm our mitochondria and cause fatigue. We'll look at some of these in the next chapter.

TTDR (TOO TIRED DIDN'T READ)

- Mitochondria make ATP by recycling it every ten seconds or so. In people with fatigue, this is reduced to once a minute. ATP is vital for our energy levels and overall health.
- Over-exercising and eating processed foods are two of the ways we can force mitochondria into overdrive, so look at how you can reduce this now.
- Undereating, overeating or yo-yo dieting puts strain on your mitochondria, but the good news is that with a consistent, nutrient-rich diet that suits your body, you can create the right environment for them to thrive.
- Hormetic stressors such as heat stress from saunas or cold stress from ice baths can all contribute to better health including higher energy levels.

SCIENCE

Different foods have different thermic effect of food values, so they take different amounts of energy to digest and absorb. Processed foods have the highest TEF values.

ONE ACTION

Make one food swap that replaces processed food with a homemade version.

ONE QUESTION

What are you doing that could be creating a bad environment for your mitochondria?

Chapter 4

What Else Could Be Wrong? *Common conditions that cause tiredness*

If you listen to your body when it whispers,
you won't have to hear it scream.

Unknown

Although mitochondrial dysfunction is at the root of many energy issues and can result from a whole range of lifestyle and environmental factors, sometimes tiredness has a very specific cause. Finding this cause is often not so easy, which is why fatigue can be so frustrating. In this chapter, we're going to investigate some of the more specific reasons for fatigue.

CAUSES OF FATIGUE SYMPTOMS

 Gut imbalances

 Food sensitivities

 Thyroid imbalances

 Autoimmune conditions

 Iron deficiency anemia

 Sleep problems

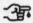 Low blood sugar

 Physiological effects of stress

(National Institutes for Quantum and Radiological Science and Technology.)

Oxidative stress

Oxidative stress can set off a chain reaction that can change the structure of cells, so long term it is not good news. In fact, oxidative stress can cause diseases such as cancer, diabetes, metabolic disorders, atherosclerosis, cardiovascular diseases and even contribute to Long Covid (Wood et al., 2021). Oxidation is the normal and necessary process of molecules transferring electrons to each other in the body. It occurs when we exercise, fight off an illness and even in the production of ATP by our old friends the mitochondria. Because the oxidation process transfers electrons, it leaves some molecules with an uneven number. These are called free radicals, and the only way to get rid of them is to neutralize them with antioxidants. Our bodies naturally make antioxidants to deal with free radicals. However, when we don't make enough, the unchecked free radicals can start to cause harm. This is called oxidative stress. One study showed that oxidative stress markers were significantly raised in people with chronic fatigue, so it could be a contributor to why you're tired (Lee et al., 2018).

Let's go even deeper into the science. Mitochondria generate around 90 per cent of cellular reactive oxygen species (ROS). Oxidative stress occurs when there is an imbalance between the ROS produced by the mitochondria, known as mtROS, and removal due to overproduction of ROS or there is a lack of antioxidants, which affects cellular components such as lipids, DNA and proteins. This is why consuming foods, such as berries, that are high in antioxidants is so important (Tirichen et al., 2021).

Metabolic dysfunction and blood sugar imbalance

In *Why We Get Sick*, Benjamin Bikman, PHD suggests that insulin resistance is the 'epidemic you've never heard of.' Insulin resistance is when cells don't respond well to insulin and therefore don't take in enough glucose from the blood. This results in the pancreas responding by producing more insulin, which can lead to Type 2 diabetes, obesity and cardiovascular disease. Research now shows there is even a Type 3 diabetes, which is linked to Alzheimer's disease and can be caused by a high fat, sugar and calorie diet (Zhao et al., 2017). The latest research suggests that people with metabolic dysfunction even have a greater rate of fatality from Covid-19.

High glucose levels also negatively impact our mitochondria. High glucose-induced mitochondrial dysfunction results with a decline of ATP production and activation of apoptotic pathway – meaning it can lead to the death of our cells (Munusamy et al., 2017).

Metabolic dysfunction has been linked to chronic fatigue and one of the key symptoms of insulin resistance is feeling excessively sleepy, especially after meals. This is because of the effect of the surge of insulin on the neurotransmitters in the brain, as well as the fact that converting sugar into fat requires a lot of energy. We'll look at how to improve metabolic function and blood sugar imbalance in Step 1 (see page 105).

Thyroid imbalances

Hormones are chemical messengers that glands send directly into the bloodstream, and they require specific nutrients to work properly. If you're not eating the right foods for your body, your hormones won't be able to do their job. Each gland plays an important role in regulating our hormones but one of the main culprits for fatigue is the butterfly-shaped gland in the neck: the thyroid.

The most common thyroid issues are hypothyroidism

(known as an under-active thyroid) and hyperthyroidism (an overactive thyroid). Hypothyroidism, in particular, is becoming increasingly more prevalent.

Different thyroid conditions have different symptoms, but can include the following as well as fatigue:

- being sensitive to cold/heat
- weight gain/loss
- constipation/diarrhoea
- depression
- muscle aches and weakness
- muscle cramps
- loss of libido
- excessive thirst

If you suspect you might have a thyroid condition, see your doctor rather than self-diagnosing and ask for a thyroid blood test.

Adrenal fatigue

The medical industry doesn't really believe that adrenal fatigue exists. Adrenal fatigue is when the adrenal glands, which sit on top of the kidneys, don't work properly. It is considered a functional issue and most of the time the underlying cause is, not surprisingly, a prolonged period of stress. The typical symptoms are:

68

- gaining weight and finding it hard to lose it, especially around the waist
- infections that last longer than normal
- shaking when under pressure
- dizziness when sitting up from a horizontal position
- inability to remember things
- feeling better shortly after meals
- feeling tired at about 9 or 10 pm but reluctant to go to bed
- needing coffee and stimulants to get going in the morning
- craving salty, fatty and protein-rich products with meat and cheese
- back or neck pain for no apparent reason
- depression
- thin, dry skin
- low blood sugar
- low body temperature
- nervousness
- heart palpitations
- digestive problems

If you think you might have adrenal fatigue you can have a test that measures your cortisol levels, but even if you don't, you can avoid adrenal fatigue by following the Five Step protocol in this book. In particular, avoiding sugar and following the sleep advice in Step 3 (see page 162) will help you avoid adrenal fatigue.

Food allergies

Food allergies are now the sixth leading cause of chronic illness in the United States, costing around $18 billion a year (ACAAI, 2022). More than 150 million Europeans suffer from chronic allergic diseases, which is set to increase to half the entire EU population by 2025 (EAACI, 2016). The reasons for this increase in food allergies aren't quite clear, but some potential culprits are the way food is produced, the chemicals and additives in food, a reduction in breastfeeding, weaning too early and changes in farming methods. It's important to remember that there are two types of food allergies: true allergies that may cause an anaphylactic shock and food intolerances.

Fatigue is a major symptom of food intolerances for two reasons. First, the immune system is trying to deal with the food sensitivity, leading to it being overworked, and second, the food is not being absorbed as readily, leading to lower micronutrient status. Allergies release chemicals known as histamines, which can cause tiredness. Certain foods, such as avocados, shellfish, dried fruit and alcohol, naturally contain histamines, so if you feel sleepy after these foods it is worth eliminating them from your diet.

Your genes

We tend to think of our genes as fixed, but did you know they have the capacity to change? Our genes are actually very sensitive to our environment, and the changes that can occur in our genes due to our lifestyle are known as epigenetics. Even the lifestyle of our parents can have an impact on our genes. In a study of epigenetics in mice, parent mice were taught to fear the smell of cherries by experiencing a tiny electric shock whenever they encountered them. Researchers found that the offspring of these mice – and even their grandchildren – showed signs of anxiety around the smell of cherries, even though they had never experienced the electric shock. I'm uncomfortable with the ethics of this research, but if the premise is true, then it suggests that changes in our body's functions could be passed down to future generations. Most interestingly, it proves that we can switch our genes on and off through our diet and lifestyle and we're not just stuck with what we're born with.

Viruses

Back in 2017, I was sitting in Richmond Park in London, admiring the river and eating an ice cream, when I noticed a fly-like creature land on my calf. I brushed it off but felt it bite me. Then I noticed this strange, circular red rash, and within weeks I felt extremely ill. I was dizzy, exhausted, weak and felt so bizarre. I thought perhaps I was having another chronic fatigue episode, but when I went to the doctor and had blood taken, he said I had the Borrelia virus, which is spread by infected ticks and can be hugely debilitating.

There I was, already suffering with my energy, only to be

told that I had Lyme disease caused by the Borrelia virus and potential co-infections too. I was prescribed antibiotics, which wreaked havoc on my body. For many weeks I couldn't stop sleeping during the day and I had completely numb arms and legs and tingling all over. It was a really frightening time as I felt I was losing control over my body. Rather than opt to take intravenous drugs in the US, which was recommended by one specialist, I decided to manage my symptoms with natural foods, herbs and supplements and, so far, things seem to have settled down.

Of course, different viruses manifest in different ways. Lyme disease typically causes a 'bullseye' rash on your body, whereas the Epstein-Barr virus may present itself in a similar way to flu. But many of them can lead to longer-term post-viral fatigue, or even CFS. More research is needed to discover why viruses sometimes stay in the system and lead to post-viral fatigue, but one theory is that viruses produce increased levels of pro-inflammatory cytokines, which promote inflammation, especially in the nervous tissue. If you suspect you have a virus, ask your GP to take blood tests to determine what type of virus it is and whether you need any treatment, such as antivirals or antibiotics.

Micronutrient deficiencies

Micronutrient deficiencies occur when the vitamin and mineral levels in your body aren't at optimal levels. Whilst there are recommended levels (known as RDAs), these are based on the population's average, which means that sometimes these levels may not be optimal for you. As we have mentioned before, if you become tired, one of the likely reasons is the imbalance between having high toxins and low micronutrients. For example, if you are drinking a lot of alcohol (a toxin), which depletes your vitamin and mineral levels, *and* you eat a nutrient-poor diet (low micronutrients), you will be low in many vitamins and minerals.

Each vitamin and mineral plays an essential role in how the body functions, but there are some likely culprits if you're experiencing fatigue:

Magnesium

Key function: generating and storing ATP and serves as a cofactor for an enzyme that repairs damaged DNA. DNA damage is a precursor to mutations that can lead to cancer and accelerate the ageing process. We also need magnesium to make and use energy

What depletes it: alcohol, smoking and some medications

Combine with: calcium for optimal absorption

Who is most at risk: people who are stressed, older adults, alcoholics and those with gastrointestinal disease due to an inability to absorb it properly

Signs: poor blood sugar metabolism, muscle cramps or soreness, eyelid twitching, fatigue and poor sleep

Iron

Key function: producing haemoglobin, a protein in red blood cells that transports oxygen to your cells

What depletes it: calcium supplements, tannins found in tea and coffee, oxalates found in spinach

Combine with: foods rich in vitamin C

Who is most at risk: childbearing women, endurance athletes, vegans or vegetarians as haem (animal) protein has a higher bioavailability than non-haem (plant) protein, those taking acid-suppressing medications, people with digestive illnesses that may impair nutrient absorption, and people with kidney failure

Signs: pale skin, chest pain, palpitations, sore tongue, weakness, cold hands and feet

B vitamins

Key function: converting the nutrients we consume from food into energy. Vitamin B is what is known as a cofactor for key metabolic processes. B6, for example, helps the body use and store energy from protein and carbohydrates in food

What depletes it: stress, alcohol, malabsorption

Combine with: magnesium

Who is most at risk: older adults and pregnant women

Signs: constipation, tingling, brain fog, numbness

Suki came to see me when she was 32. She had given birth to her baby girl 6 months earlier and was feeling exhausted and depleted. Suki had had a traumatic birth – she required a blood transfusion and had lost a lot of blood. She was breastfeeding and didn't have time to make proper nutrient-dense meals, instead grabbing any snack that was available. This was usually a high-carbohydrate and high-sugar cereal bar. She was feeling emotional and was experiencing aches and pains.

I requested Suki see her doctor to assess her iron levels and test her thyroid. In the meantime, as iron levels post-birth can take a year to restore, I decided to include lots of iron-rich haem (animal) and non-haem (plant) foods into her diet. This included grass-fed beef, spinach and liver (Suki didn't like liver much, so we chopped it up into homemade spaghetti bolognese and cottage pie), tofu and dried apricots. To facilitate the absorption of iron, we included vitamin C-rich foods, such as red and yellow peppers, kale, kiwis and broccoli. I prescribed her a good multivitamin specifically formulated to support breastfeeding and suggested she ate little and often, with protein in every meal and snack. We ensured she was drinking enough water. I advised her to have a water bottle and nuts and seeds with her at all times, so she could remain properly hydrated and have an immediate protein-rich, healthy snack readily available to balance her blood sugar levels. We introduced 30 minutes every day of uninterrupted time for her so she could take a bath, go for a walk or read a book.

In her follow-up, Suki said she felt much better. As suspected, when the results came back from the doctor her iron levels were lower than the optimal ranges and she was anaemic, so we worked even harder to restore her iron. This was like a domino effect: because Suki had more energy, she started cooking for herself and her family again, which further improved her energy as the food was more nutrient dense.

Sometimes, like Suki, there is a specific cause of your fatigue, and looking at your other symptoms can often give you clues about what that could be. Think of yourself as a detective, digging deep into the evidence to build a picture of what's going on. Keeping a journal or using a tracker of your symptoms, your stress and energy levels and the foods you eat can be a good way to keep track of your body's patterns. If you suspect a thyroid issue or a virus such as Lyme disease, see your doctor, take your symptom tracker so you don't forget anything and ask for blood tests. Make sure you ask for a copy of your results so you can look at the ranges. Many people who are unwell still fall within the normal ranges.

Questions you may want to ask your doctor are:

- What blood tests can I have?
- What other blood tests that aren't routinely given may be useful here?
- What is the plan of action to tackle this?
- When shall I return for my follow-up?
- Can you recommend any other nutrition or lifestyle interventions or a referral that may be helpful here?

Remember not to feel silly, or that your tiredness is trivial. It is very real for you and it isn't normal. Try and get your doctor to understand the full picture of your symptoms and not withhold anything that may be useful so they can properly advise the next steps.

TTDR (TOO TIRED DIDN'T READ)

- Oxidative stress is the imbalance of free radicals and antioxidants and is a major cause of fatigue.
- Blood sugar imbalance can lead to metabolic dysfunction, which not only increases the risk of diabetes and cardiovascular disease, but can cause long-term fatigue.
- Thyroid disorders are on the rise. Symptoms include excessive thirst, tiredness, weight loss or gain and sensitivity to heat or cold.
- Symptoms of adrenal fatigue include weight gain, dizziness and difficulty getting up in the morning.
- Food intolerances cause fatigue by reducing absorption and putting strain on the immune system.
- Viruses such as Epstein-Barr and Lyme disease can trigger chronic fatigue. If you think you have been infected, see your doctor.

SCIENCE

One study showed that oxidative stress markers were significantly raised in people with chronic fatigue, so it could be a contributor to why you're tired (Lee et al., 2018).

ONE ACTION

Keep a diary of your symptoms and check if any of them fit with any of the conditions in this chapter.

ONE QUESTION

Which foods trigger a bad reaction after eating them?

Chapter 5

Why Don't Doctors Have All the Answers?
The roles of traditional and functional medicine

> The doctor of the future will give no medicine
> but will interest his patients in the care of the
> human frame, in diet and in the cause and
> prevention of disease.
>
> Thomas Edison

Many of my clients come to me because after multiple trips to their doctor and every blood test under the sun – all of which have come back normal – they still don't know what's wrong. Some of them have even been prescribed treatments like antibiotics, antidepressants or IBS medication, and yet their symptoms still remain.

One such client was Peter. When Peter came to see me, I could see straight away that he had bad eczema on his eyelids.

He told me that it was also on his legs, and although the steroid cream his doctor had prescribed had worked initially, the itching and flaking were now worse than ever. Peter worked in the City in finance and he admitted that his job was fairly stressful, but he said that generally his mood was good, he felt positive and had a lot of good things going on in his life. However, his skin was telling me a different story.

I decided to question Peter a bit more about his diet and his medical history. He told me that he ate out on average three times a week and often drank around 25 units a week of wine and beer. His diet was good when his wife cooked for him at home, but when he ate out he usually opted for pizza or a cheeseburger and fries. When I asked about his birth and early childhood, Peter said that he had been delivered by caesarean section and his mother had struggled to breastfeed. He said his skin was often worse during the week when he wasn't at home.

I explained to Peter that, although the steroid cream had provided a short-term solution to his eczema, it wasn't tackling the root cause. After more thorough investigations, I felt that the real cause was a combination of stress, dairy intolerance and dysbiosis in his gut, which was in turn affecting the skin–gut axis. The plan I put together included adding lots of nourishing probiotic foods into his diet to improve his gut microbiome and switching dairy for nut milks, nut cheese and coconut yoghurt. The plan focused on cutting down on sugar as it can be a risk factor for eczema. We included a probiotic supplement specifically formulated to tackle eczema and incorporated stress reduction techniques, such as mindfulness and tai chi. We removed any toiletry products that may have been producing an allergic response and replaced them with toxin-free versions. He agreed to cut down on alcohol.

By the time Peter's follow-up came around his skin had cleared up and his energy levels had improved. In fact, he said he hadn't realized how stressed he had become.

Why wasn't Peter's doctor able to find out what was wrong? First, let me start by saying that traditional medicine has a vital role to play in treating ill health, including fatigue. This is because doctors can:

- rule out serious health conditions
- perform blood tests and diagnose deficiencies
- check for hormone imbalances, for example in your thyroid
- diagnose autoimmune conditions or viruses, such as Lyme disease

However, if everything your doctor looks at comes back as normal, it's time for a different approach. You need to take matters into your own hands. This is because, while some doctors might look at things more holistically, it's generally unrealistic to expect a general practitioner to take into account your past, your current lifestyle, your mental, emotional, spiritual and psychological state and everything you've been eating and drinking, all in a ten-minute appointment. So, just as the person at the centre of your energy is you, the person responsible for finding out why you're tired is also . . . you.

What's the alternative?

What is functional medicine and how does it work? Functional medicine is different to western medicine in that it seeks to find the root cause of the symptoms experienced. It is an evidence-based approach to healthcare, which believes we are all biochemically unique, hence why taking a personalized, tailored approach is far more effective in the long term. It is holistic and patient-centred, believing at its core that health is not just about the absence of disease, there is so much more to it than that.

> Functional medicine is a disruptive technology
> that will overthrow the tyranny of the diagnosis.
>
> Jeffrey Bland, PhD

Functional medicine works by identifying the root cause of what's wrong with you. Rather than being disease-centred – in other words, focused on treating your symptoms – it's patient-centred, meaning it seeks to treat the whole person. So, while traditional western medicine wants to ascertain what's wrong with you, functional medicine wants to know why.

The key premise of functional medicine is that it views all the body's systems as interconnected – each having an impact on the other. Genes, the environment, nutrition and lifestyle are all taken into consideration to create a personalized solution.

This is what we need to do to get to the root cause of your fatigue because, just as the reason you are tired will be unique to you, the solution to your tiredness needs to be tailored to you and your unique biochemistry.

For example, your fatigue could be due to something out of kilter in the nervous system, the endocrine system or the musculoskeletal, gastrointestinal, immune or cardiovascular systems – or even a combination of them all. In functional medicine no system is overlooked, and every aspect of your health is explored in depth via a full consultation.

TRADITIONAL VS FUNCTIONAL MEDICINE

Traditional medicine is:
- disease-centred
- preventative
- one-size-fits-all

Functional medicine is:
- patient-centred
- holistic
- tailored to your unique biochemistry

Functional medicine operates on the basis that we are complex human beings with complex systems that all interact. Therefore, your tiredness is not likely to be caused by just one problem, but by a 'perfect storm' of many factors. These can be split into antecedents, mediators and triggers:

Antecedents
Your genetic disposition towards the disease.

Mediators
Anything that may contribute to the disease over a period of time, such as a high-sugar diet, anxiety or stress.

Triggers
Any events that could have caused the onset, such as a virus or a traumatic event.

When should we switch to a more functional approach to fixing our fatigue? The answer is that it's never too early to make positive changes to your diet and lifestyle, but first let's explore the role of your doctor and how functional medicine can work with conventional medicine.

The role of your doctor

If you haven't already, the first thing to do when exploring why you're tired is to visit your doctor. Explain your symptoms, ideally with the help of a symptom diary, and ask for a full set of blood tests. Blood testing can be a minefield and knowing which tests to start off with can feel daunting, especially because there isn't a specific test to measure your energy levels. However, the following tests are a good place to start:

USEFUL TESTS

Full blood count
White blood cell (WBC) count, also known as leukocytes, red blood cell (RBC) count and iron.

Specific iron markers
Serum ferritin, total/serum iron, total/transferrin iron binding capacity, transferrin saturation to diagnose iron deficiency or iron overload and anaemia.

Thyroid test
TSH, T4, T3 and thyroid antibodies (TPO, Tg, TSH) to assess any hormonal or thyroid dysregulation, such as hypothyroidism or autoimmunity.

Blood glucose tests
HbA1c to monitor average blood glucose levels, fasting glucose and glucose tolerance to measure glucose levels in the blood and check for diabetes.

Urine test
To test for infections, including UTIs.

Stool test
To see if there is blood, bacteria, yeasts or parasites.

Cholesterol test
Total cholesterol, low-density lipoprotein (LDL) cholesterol ('bad' cholesterol), high-density lipoprotein (HDL) cholesterol ('good' cholesterol) to assess build-up of fatty deposits in the arteries.

Triglycerides
Measures the amount of triglycerides or fat in the blood. High triglycerides can be a sign of metabolic syndrome.

Blood pressure
To check if you have high or low blood pressure.

CRP (C-reactive protein)
To assess for the presence of inflammation and its severity.

ESR (Erythrocyte sedimentation rate)
To detect and monitor the activity of inflammation.

Your doctor might ask you what colour your urine normally is, or if you have had blood or mucus in your stools, so keep checking these so you can provide them with the correct information. These charts are a good way of knowing which type you are:

How to read your pee

URINE COLOUR CHART

Over hydrated	No color
Good	Pale straw yellow
Fair	Translucent yellow
Lightly dehydrated	Dark yellow
Dehydrated	Amber
Very dehydrated	Burnt orange
Severely dehydrated	Red

How to read your poo

STOOL TYPES AND WHAT THEY MEAN

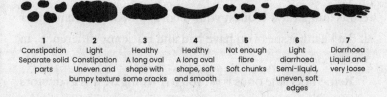

1	2	3	4	5	6	7
Constipation Separate solid parts	Light Constipation Uneven and bumpy texture	Healthy A long oval shape with some cracks	Healthy A long oval shape, soft and smooth	Not enough fibre Soft chunks	Light diarrhoea Semi-liquid, uneven, soft edges	Diarrhoea Liquid and very loose

Ideally, your urine will be a pale straw colour and your stools type 3 or 4 on the Stool Chart.

As the doctors' panel – bloodwork – only paints part of the picture, seeing a nutritionist will provide a more comprehensive overview of what may be going on as more tests can be given. However, in functional medicine we wouldn't stop there. If you have a deficiency there is often a reason underlying that deficiency, so it's important to follow the questions in the next section to get to the real root of your symptoms.

One of the big problems with blood tests is your results might be in the range of normal, but the problem with this is what 'normal' represents. In traditional blood tests, the normal reference ranges provided are based on the average of the population – many of whom might be feeling as poorly as you are but haven't had anything diagnosed. That's why it's important to discuss the ranges with your doctor and find out what's *optimal* rather than just within normal range. One way to do this is to have your blood tested regularly so you know what's normal for you and you can then spot any downward trends.

Everyone has a different genetic make up, which requires a different level of micronutrients, so what's optimal for one person might not be sufficient for another. Keep track of your results and always request your records so you can remember all the health issues you have had and track any differences in your bloods.

Remember: the onus is on you to investigate this as doctors

simply cannot do this for all their clients and you can get more comprehensive testing via a reputable nutritionist.

Red flags

Another important role your doctor can play is to identify any 'red flags' that might indicate an acute and/or serious condition. If in conjunction with your fatigue you're experiencing any of the symptoms below, speak to your doctor immediately:

- blood in sputum, vomit, urine, semen or stools (blood can sometimes be hidden)
- vomit containing 'coffee grounds'
- severe, unremitting bone pain
- low back pain associated with difficulty urinating and defecating, and/or pain/altered sensation down both legs
- black, tarry stools
- significant vaginal bleeding that is not associated with menstruation
- persistent vomiting and/or diarrhoea
- persistent dry cough
- unexplained weight loss not associated with a weight-loss programme (1.5kg/3lb or more per week)
- difficulty swallowing
- a skin lesion (evolving size, shape, colour, bleeding, itching, pain)

- a change in bowel habits, often with rectal bleeding
- drenching night sweats (this can be common post-birth)
- unexplained swelling or lumps
- unexplained fever, particularly if persistent or recurrent
- excessive urination and increased thirst
- thunderclap headache (explosive onset of a new headache)
- worsening morning headaches that are exacerbated by movement

TOP TIP 🖉

If something has been niggling at you or bothering you, don't wait to get it checked out. If you need quick advice, call 111. Dr Google isn't advisable if you aren't an experienced medical practitioner.

Unravelling your symptoms

Once you've been to the doctor, had some blood tests and discounted any underlying health issues raised by the red flags, now is the time to turn to functional medicine to get to the root of why you're tired.

Time after time I meet people in my clinic who have received normal blood results and yet still have ongoing symptoms they can't get rid of. I've personally experienced it. I remember going to my GP many times. While my iron would be low or my white blood cells out of range, most of my results would be fine. Yet I still felt terrible. This lack of answers made me feel despondent – or that perhaps I was overreacting or being a hypochondriac. It can be incredibly frustrating, but the key thing here is not to give up. Keep digging, exploring and tweaking your lifestyle, because life is not fun if you don't feel good.

So, where do we start with a more functional medicine approach to your health? Well, most functional medicine practitioners start with what we call the kaleidoscope of your health. This is known as your exposome.

Before we are even born, and throughout our lives, we are exposed to a number of different factors. The sum total of these makes up our exposome. This overall picture of our health includes the food we eat, the environmental toxins we are exposed to and even our thoughts and emotions – all of which can affect our energy. In other words, the exposome is the build-up of personal and external environmental stressors combined with the subsequent biological responses that make us feel like we do.

There are three areas within the exposome – the personal, external and biological responses. You can see from the diagram over the page how they're all separate but how they overlap with each other too.

THE EXPOSOME

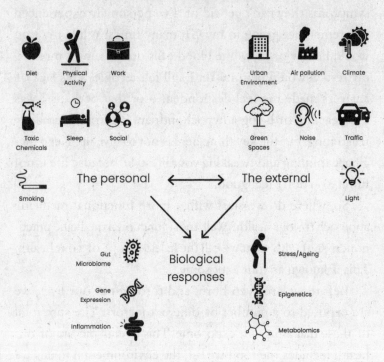

Diet · Physical Activity · Work · Urban Environment · Air pollution · Climate

Toxic Chemicals · Sleep · Social · Green Spaces · Noise · Traffic

The personal ⟷ The external

Smoking · Light

Gut Microbiome · Biological responses · Stress/Ageing

Gene Expression · Epigenetics

Inflammation · Metabolomics

The personal exposome

What you eat, how you choose to move, your choice of job and career, the chemicals you expose yourself to knowingly or unknowingly, the quality and quantity of your sleep, your connections and relationships and whether you smoke all have a huge impact on your health. This personal exposome affects your genes, your gut microbiome, how quickly you age and how inflamed your body becomes. To some extent, you have control over your personal exposome. Armed with this information, you have the power to make changes so you don't have to feel like this forever.

On a personal level, I believe that following the wrong career path for years contributed to making me unwell. My mind and body were both trying to tell me that they weren't enjoying the high pressure, stress and career incompatibility, yet I kept drowning out the signals with late nights, poor food choices, alcohol and inconsistent sleep. It was only when I looked at it all in relation to the other issues that I could see what was making me chronically tired.

To start to uncover what might be making up your personal exposome, ask yourself these 15 questions:

YOUR PERSONAL EXPOSOME FINDING OUT THE ROOT CAUSE

1. When were you last fit and well?
2. What has changed since then? Did anything specific happen?
3. How did you come to recognize your low energy?
4. What are your primary current stressors? List the top three.
5. How can these stressors be alleviated before changing your lifestyle?

Your personal energy

6. When do you have the least amount of energy and why?

7. What gives you energy? When do you feel full of energy?

8. What takes your energy away/what are your energy leaks?

9. Do you feel fulfilled and content? If not, why not?

10. What causes fatigue, what makes it worse and what relieves it?

How you feel day-to-day

11. How would you describe your other symptoms?

12. How much effort does it take to get going in the morning?

13. What is the quality of your sleep? Does a good night's sleep relieve your fatigue?

14. How much exercise can you sustain, and what happens afterwards?

15. Is there a time of day or month when your fatigue is worse?

If you would like to write your answers down please turn to the notes pages on p.231

The external exposome

These days we are exposed to many toxic substances – in our food, water and air – and it's becoming increasingly important that we're able to detoxify these from our bodies. Low-level toxicity is a silent contributor to fatigue and many other illnesses. In fact, environmental risk factors contribute to 70–90 per cent of all disease – including cancers (Anand et al., 2008). Before we throw up our hands in horror at this, we should find it encouraging – it means there are things we can do to decrease our risk of serious disease.

So, how can we measure our exposure to harmful toxins? If you have the money, you could commission private blood and urine tests, but if not, then the 10 questions below will give you a good idea of your environmental, chemical and pollution risk profile:

Your environmental, chemical and pollution risk profile	
Do you live in a city or by a busy road?	Y/N
Do you spend 2 hours a week or more in traffic?	Y/N
Do you exercise by a busy road?	Y/N
Do you smoke?	Y/N
Do you work or live in a smoky atmosphere?	Y/N
Does your work entail handling toxic substances such as herbicides or chemicals?	Y/N
Do you spend much time in front of a VDU?	Y/N
Do you use chemical cleaning products?	Y/N
Do you use chemicals in your makeup and toiletries?	Y/N
Do you have mould in your home?	Y/N

Add up your total number of Y. If it's between 0–3 = low risk, 3–6 = medium risk and 6–10 = high risk (see Step 2 Support Your Gut on page 144 for ideas on what to do if you get a high-risk score).

Biological responses

As we learnt in Chapter 4 (see page 70), our genes can be 'switched on' or 'switched off' by environmental factors – otherwise known as epigenetics. This is why the biological responses circle overlaps the other two circles in the exposome. So, you might be predisposed to diabetes, but through nutrition and lifestyle choices you can switch this gene off to stop it becoming defective or mutating.

Our biological responses include our gut microbiome. In fact, I would go as far as to say that the majority of cases of fatigue I see in my clinic are down to an imbalance in the bacteria in the gut known as gut dysbiosis. And gut dysbiosis can cause other conditions too. Here are a few more common health conditions that are associated with the microbiome (Williams et al., 2018):

- acne
- antibiotic-associated diarrhoea
- asthma/allergies
- autism
- autoimmune diseases

- dental cavities
- depression and anxiety
- diabetes
- eczema
- gastric ulcers
- hardening of the arteries
- inflammatory bowel diseases
- malnutrition
- obesity

If you have one or many of these symptoms, you will benefit from some gut support, which is why Step 2 (see page 144) in the second half of this book is all to do with the microbiome.

Some studies have found that there are specific bacteria in the gut that seem to correlate with chronic fatigue. In one 2017 study, researchers analysed faecal samples from 50 people with chronic fatigue syndrome and 50 healthy people. The differences in the levels of six particular types of gut bacteria – Faecalibacterium, Roseburia, Dorea, Coprococcus, Clostridium, Ruminococcus and Coprobacillu – correlated so strongly with CFS that they could predict which people had the condition just from the bacteria in their gut (Mishra et al., 2017). This proves not just how much good bacteria you need to have in your gut, but the specific type of bacteria.

So, what's gone so wrong with our gut to make it out of balance and cause us fatigue and other symptoms? Because the gut is so sensitive and clever, there are many factors that can influence it.

Early life

The makeup of the gut microbiome starts *in utero*. The paediatric microbiome has been studied extensively in recent years and research has shown that the 'critical window' of gut development is the time between conception and the first year of life. This is when the microbiome is most sensitive to environmental factors. For this reason, the mother's microbiome and diet can play a role in determining the health of the gut (Gaufin et al., 2018). Early-life environmental exposures can also affect the immune system, putting it into a hypersensitive or hyper inflammatory state (Stiemsma and Michels, 2018). The great news is that the gut is adaptable – it has the capacity to change. If you think your energy has always been poor, and whilst I appreciate it is not always possible, talk to your mother about her microbiome, gut and diet. Find out how you were born and whether you were breastfed or bottle-fed. All these seemingly trivial questions are important to complete the full health picture of you.

Antibiotics

Antibiotics are essential in treating serious bacterial infections like meningitis, pneumonia, sepsis and many others. However, they aren't suitable for coughs, earache and sore throats but increasingly are being given out for these illnesses. As a result, antibiotic resistance and antibiotic misuse is on the increase and in many instances antibiotics just don't work. According to many experts, we are on the precipice of a post-antibiotic apocalypse, with serious consequences for our health.

On top of that, antibiotics wreak havoc on the gut because they kill off many of the good bacteria along with the harmful ones they're trying to treat. After each course of antibiotics, the gut takes time to repair – sometimes many months. Excessive use of antibiotics, especially in early childhood, can contribute to gut dysbiosis later in life. There are many natural antibiotics, such as garlic, manuka honey, ginger, echinacea, oregano, goldenseal and cloves, which can be tried if the doctor agrees that antibiotics don't have to be the first port of call and you would like some additional natural support. If you are on any medication, it is always best to check that if you take something else, even if it's natural, that there isn't a drug/nutrient interaction, which may impact the effectiveness of the medication or cause an unwanted side effect.

I hope in the future that seeing a nutritionist is just as common and deemed as important as going to the doctor. That nutritionists and doctors sit side-by-side in practice to develop a co-joined bespoke protocol for every client. Looking for the underlying root cause and reviewing the whole person – from birth to the current day – is the only way to paint a comprehensive picture of your health. That's why the Five Step plan we're going to look at now deals with all aspects of your exposome, tackling each area in turn so you can truly fix your tiredness.

TTDR (TOO TIRED DIDN'T READ)

- Your doctor plays a fundamental role in discovering why you're tired.
- Functional medicine looks at the whole picture and how your bodily systems interact.
- Your exposome is made up of the environmental factors that contribute to disease outcomes.
- Your personal exposome is made up of your work, sleep, social activity, exercise and diet.
- Your external exposome is your exposure to toxins and harmful chemicals from toiletries, pollution, cleaning products and moulds.
- Your biological responses are the way your genes switch on and off, how you age, your gut microbiome and how your body handles inflammation.
- Functional medicine doesn't just look at your current lifestyle but factors from pre-birth and childhood, too.

SCIENCE

Environmental risk factors contribute to 70–90 per cent of all disease risk. Only 10 per cent are genetic factors.

ONE ACTION

If you haven't already, go to your doctor and request blood tests to rule out underlying conditions that could be causing your fatigue.

ONE QUESTION

Is there anything from your past that might give you clues about why you're tired now?

Part 2

Five Steps to Feeling Less Tired

Step 1

Fuel Your Body
Eating for energy

> If you get the inside right, the outside will fall
> into place. Primary reality is within; secondary
> reality without.
>
> Eckhart Tolle

When I was in my twenties, I thought my diet was pretty healthy. I'd have a bowl of tinned tomato soup with wholemeal bread for lunch and think that was a good meal. I thought a gyoza noodle bowl or tuna fishcakes with salad bought from a nice super-market meant I was eating well. Was I wrong? Well, yes and no.

The truth is, there's nothing 'wrong' with those meals. In fact, the first thing I want to say is that we need to stop thinking about certain foods or meals as 'good' or 'bad'. That isn't a healthy way to think, and it's why we're not going to talk about calories, fat intake, demon carbs or 'good' or 'bad' foods for even one second in this first step to fixing your fatigue. Instead, I want us to focus on the kind of long-term nutrition that can change the way you feel and, more specifically, give you bags more energy.

You might wonder how much of a difference food really makes. After all, you've eaten this way for years and felt OK. Does food really make that much of a difference? I am here to tell you that it does. Over the long term, a nutrient-poor diet will always catch up with you. It might not be immediate – in fact, you might have been getting away with it for years – but at some point, you will start to feel a little 'off'. Your digestion might suffer, you might get more coughs and colds, or you might start to feel increasingly tired.

Think back to Chapter 3 (see page 51) and our lovely little mitochondria. You'll remember that these power stations inside our cells are fuelled by what we put in our bodies – in other words, our food. Everything we eat, digest and absorb determines how well our chemical reactions work within our body, specifically our cells. This is why fad diets are so damaging: they cause our bodies to lack the nutrients needed for the processes it relies on.

So, the important thing to remember as we take our first step to fixing our fatigue is that it's not how *much* we put in our bodies that matters, but how nutritious it is. That's why to really change the way we feel about food we need to stop focusing on dieting and start focusing on what I call BIG nutrition.

Why BIG?

Our food is fuel for our bodies and, as Eckhart Tolle said, if you get the inside right, the outside will fall into place. So, all our meals should be BIG – that is, focused on:

B = **Brain**
I = **Immunity**
G = **Gut**

Let's look at each of the BIG systems in turn:

Brain

As we learnt in Chapter 1 (see page 33), your brain uses up 20 per cent of your overall energy. It's vital that it has the right nutrients to work optimally and protect your mental health. You might know that serotonin is the 'happy' hormone that makes us sleep and regulates our mood, but did you know that about 90 per cent of serotonin is made in the gut, not the brain? What you eat really does affect how you think and feel, as well as how well rested you are. When serotonin is low, it can affect wellbeing and cause anxiety and depression, as well as fatigue.

Feeding your brain the right foods can really help, especially if you are feeling cognitively tired. Some top brain foods are:

- berries – blueberries, raspberries, strawberries
- good fats – olives, olive oil, avocado, avocado oil
- oily fish – salmon, mackerel, herring
- fermented foods – sauerkraut, kefir, kombucha, miso
- leafy greens – spinach, kale, cabbage
- hydrating foods – melons, cucumbers, kiwi, pineapple

- eggs
- dark foods – black beans, purple sprouting broccoli, 80% dark chocolate
- tryptophan-containing foods – oats, bananas, turkey

TOP TIP 🖉

Combine tryptophan-rich foods with 25–30 grams of complex carbohydrates (found in whole grains, legumes and vegetables) to ensure they cross the blood–brain barrier. For example, combine nuts (tryptophan rich) and oats (complex carbohydrate) or salmon (tryptophan rich) or turkey (tryptophan rich) and brown rice (complex carbohydrate). Be aware tryptophan conversion to serotonin can be impaired by dysbiosis – an imbalance in the gut – deficiency of iron, B6 and a niacin derivative called THB. Inflammation in the central nervous system can prevent tryptophan conversion to serotonin and low oestrogen (menopause) may also lead to reduced levels and also lower melatonin, this being one factor in poor sleep quality in perimenopause and menopause.

Immune system

Your immune system determines how well you will fight off infections and pathologies – even more important in times of a pandemic. We have two levels of immune system: our innate immune system and our adaptive immune system.

Our innate immune system is our natural first line of defence. It's made up of things like the skin, which is our primary barrier, and our mucous membranes that line our lungs, mouth, nose and eyelids. It is quick to respond to an invader.

In the adaptive immune system we have cells called B and T cells. T cells are memory cells – they recognize what invader has invaded and use the right weapon to destroy it. B cells create antibodies and markers so that the invader is more recognizable. The adaptive immune system in the long term will serve us better in fighting infection because it learns how to develop a specific response to a pathogen.

So how can we 'boost' our immune system? The answer is we can't, and if any company is selling you products that claim to do this, avoid them like the plague. What we can do is introduce immune-supporting foods, herbs and supplements into our everyday diet. The immune system is generally asleep until triggered multiple times into a state of increased alertness and activity by molecular signals we either consume or are produced by our bodies. These include:

- red peppers
- manuka honey

- garlic
- carrots
- chillies
- ginger
- yoghurt
- leafy greens
- sweet potatoes
- mushrooms
- Brazil nuts
- turmeric

TOP TIP

Have 1–2 spoonfuls of raw or local honey from your area containing methylglyoxal (MGO) a day to increase your immunity and help prevent or soothe colds and coughs. MGO is beneficial due to its high antibacterial properties. Local pollen can help strengthen your immune system and support pollen allergies. It has good antimicrobial properties too. Turn to the Resources pages at the back of the book to see where you can source local honey from.

Gut

We now know that what happens in the gut affects almost every part of the body, including our energy levels. We'll learn specifically how to support the gut in Step 2 (see page 144), but here are some top gut foods to get you started:

- sauerkraut
- kimchi
- yoghurt
- kefir
- miso
- sourdough
- almonds
- olive oil
- kombucha

I am not a perfect eater and neither do I aspire to be, but I try 80 per cent of the time to follow the BIG philosophy. You can do this too, by getting into the habit of thinking how you can make each meal as nutritionally dense as possible in a way that will support your brain, immune and gut health. This will vary from person to person. You may be someone who thrives on more healthy fats and a lower carbohydrate diet. Or you might prefer a high carbohydrate, lower fat diet. The important thing is to experiment and get creative to find out what type of lifestyle feels good for you. The clue to knowing whether it is working for you is in how you feel after incorporating BIG changes. So, here's how you should feel when you eat BIG:

- energized
- no stomach pains or bloating
- clear skin
- reduced cravings for carbohydrates and sugar
- stable energy levels
- consistent mood

How to build a BIG plate

So, how do we start to make BIG changes to our diet? Well, the first thing I want you to know is that we are not going to take anything away. Sounds crazy? Maybe. Of course, if you're eating lots of processed food then we want to aim to reduce that over time and replace it with more nutritious choices, but the most important goal in this step isn't to cut foods out but to *add them in*.

To show you what I mean, let's take another look at my meal of tinned tomato soup and wholemeal bread at the start of this step. It's not an unhealthy meal, but it's not BIG. Here's why:

- The shop-bought tomato soup lacks the vitamins and minerals you'd get in a homemade version because it's been processed – in other words,

many of the nutrients have been lost through the manufacturing process.
- The meal doesn't contain any real protein source, so will not increase the feeling of fullness, possibly causing me to consume sugary snacks later on.
- Along with the lack of protein, the brown bread will raise blood sugar levels as it is a medium-to-high glycaemic index food.

So, you can see how even though it's not a *bad* meal, it isn't as nutritious as it could be. So, what could we add to this meal to make it BIG? Here are some ideas:

- Make the soup homemade – and don't just use tomatoes. Add carrot, peppers or squash to increase the variety of vegetables.
- Add some protein, such as chickpeas or beans, or add tuna to the bread.
- Sprinkle some healthy fat-containing seeds on the soup.
- Swap the bread for rye bread or sourdough, which contain prebiotics.

Or what about the gyoza meal? Again, there's nothing wrong with it, but we can easily do a few additions to make it BIG:

- Buy or make good-quality bone broth instead of shop-bought. You could use a leftover chicken carcass from a roast dinner to create yours.

- Add chicken and a boiled egg for protein.
- Add green leafy veg for vitamins and minerals.
- Swap the noodles for brown rice noodles if gluten is a trigger.

From this I hope you can see that eating BIG isn't about going on a diet or denying yourself delicious food. In fact, it's not about taking things away at all, but *adding* nutritious foods so that everything you eat is as nutritionally dense as possible.

We can do this by building each plate of food around the BIG formula below:

> Protein + healthy fats + complex carbs +
> antioxidants and micronutrients

Note: Not every meal and snack you have needs a complex carb, but you can add them in for at least one meal a day.

Protein

So, start off with some form of protein. This could be:

- grass-fed beef
- chicken

- SMASH fish that are high in Omega 3 – Sardines, Mackerel, Anchovies, Salmon and Herring. Though be careful of consuming too much high-mercury (a neurotoxin) fish like tuna and swordfish. Limit fish like tuna and swordfish to twice a week
- tofu
- tempeh
- seitan
- vegetarian mince

Healthy fats

Now add a source of healthy fat. This could be:

- olive oil
- coconut oil
- nuts, such as almonds, macadamia nuts and walnuts
- seeds, such as linseeds, pumpkin seeds, flaxseed, chia seeds
- SMASH fish (Sardines, Mackerel, Anchovies, Salmon and Herring)
- avocados
- whole eggs

Complex carbs

Now you can opt to add a complex, low-GI carbohydrate, such as:

- sweet potatoes
- beans, such as kidney, butter beans or black beans
- oats
- chickpeas
- lentils
- brown rice

While white potatoes and white rice are still nutritious and there's no need to eliminate them from your diet, they just don't contain as many nutrients as their complex cousins above and they might raise your blood sugar more quickly.

Antioxidants and micronutrients

Finally, add colourful ingredients that contain antioxidants and micronutrients, such as spices, herbs, fruit and vegetables. These protect against oxidative stress and add vital vitamins and minerals to your diet. Some examples are:

- blueberries
- strawberries
- broccoli
- peppers (all colours)
- cauliflower
- leafy greens

Nutrient 'toppers'

TOP TIP 🖊

Get some glass jars and sticky labels, pick a cupboard and label all your nutrient toppers. I tend to get them out first thing in the morning so my partner and I can add whatever we fancy. This way, you will never forget to add the extra layer of nutrients to your food if they are in sight and readily available.

If you've been on a diet or weight-loss programme for a while, eating BIG might be hard to get your head around, but it's important to switch your focus here. Eating healthily isn't about cutting core food groups and nutrients out or measuring calories. It's about adding additional nutrients into whatever you are eating. A quick and easy way to do this without feeling like you're eating too many calories is to 'top' your meals with added ingredients to increase their nutritional value. Some of the things on the list below might not sound nice, but in many cases they taste better than they look. Find the ones you like and start experimenting with topping your meals:

- flaxseed
- linseeds

- pumpkin seeds
- coconut flakes
- berries – fresh and dried, such as goji
- toasted tree nuts, such as cashews, pecans, pistachios and almonds
- black and white sesame seeds
- pine nuts
- olive oil
- pickled carrot
- ginger
- kimchi
- sauerkraut
- sprouted mung beans
- nori flakes
- broccoli sprouts

TOP TIP ✏️

Eating a handful of almonds a day improves gut health by increasing butyrate, a short-chain fatty acid that acts as a power source for cells in the colon. They regulate absorption of other nutrients in the gut and help balance the immune system. (Kings College London, 2022)

You can never have too many of these on your plate. Ideally, focus on green leafy vegetables for their high magnesium and liver supportive properties. Try to eat seasonally with as much diversity as possible and be experimental with flavourings and cooking methods to avoid getting bored.

A perfect example of how adding foods to your diet can fix your fatigue was Howard. Howard was 37 and a dedicated athlete, but he came to my clinic saying he didn't feel energized enough for his training. He was presenting with fatigue, diarrhoea, poor sleep, muscle cramps and joint stiffness. When we delved into his case history and diet, we realized that his diet was severely lacking in micronutrients. It was high in carbohydrates because that's what Howard thought he needed to give him energy to train, but it lacked protein and fibre. Howard relied on processed snacks like high-sugar training bars to keep him going throughout the day.

Instead of telling Howard to cut a whole load of foods out, we started by adding more nutrients to his diet. Howard liked a fry-up on a Sunday morning, so we decided he would add in some roasted tomatoes, roasted broccoli and spinach sautéed in garlic and oil. He also added some homemade Boston baked beans and before he knew it, he'd turned a low-nutrient meal into a nutrient-dense breakfast of champions. We increased Howard's intake of legumes and pulses to boost the fibre in his diet and added in some homemade snacks in the form of energy bars and balls, sourdough toast, carrots and hummus and apple and nut butter with seeds and protein smoothies. Before long, Howard didn't need the sugary energy bars and within a few weeks he felt more energized – just by adding foods *into* his diet.

Don't know what to eat? Here are the most nutritionally dense foods. Try adding a different one of these ingredients to your meals every day and before you know it, you'll be eating 30 nutrient-dense foods across your month.

1. seaweeds
2. liver (beef and chicken)
3. leafy greens, like kale, spring greens, spinach, watercress, dandelion greens and rocket
4. broccoli, cauliflower and other cruciferous veggies, like cabbage or Brussels sprouts
5. exotic berries, like acai and goji
6. red, yellow, green and orange peppers
7. carrots and parsnips
8. garlic
9. parsley, coriander, basil and other herbs
10. berries, like blueberries, raspberries and blackberries
11. asparagus
12. beets
13. wild salmon and sardines
14. bone broth
15. grass-fed beef
16. green beans
17. egg yolks

18. pumpkin
19. lentils
20. artichokes
21. tomatoes
22. wild mushrooms
23. seeds, like pumpkin, sunflower, chia and flax
24. raw cheese and kefir
25. sweet potatoes
26. black beans
27. wild rice
28. yoghurt
29. cacao
30. avocado

(Taken from Dr Axe)

TOP TIP ✏️

Just including more of these highly nutritious foods into your diet is a good start. If you don't like liver, you can buy liver capsules from reputable companies and sprinkle the contents into your spaghetti bolognese. Stir-fry diced Brussels sprouts with garlic and ginger; create a bone-broth stock using your chicken bones; roast broccoli and cauliflower and add seaweed flakes to salads.

QUICK RECIPE COMBINATIONS USING THE PREVIOUS FOODS

Sweet potato + avocado + tomatoes + sunflower seeds + salmon = **baked potato and salmon**

Black beans + wild rice + yoghurt + avocado + tomato salsa = **black bean chilli**

Grass-fed beef + sweet potato chips and/or parsnip chips + green beans = **steak and chips**

Kefir yoghurt + berries + seeds = **breakfast bowl**

Grass-fed beef and/or lentils + cacao (dark chocolate 70%) + tomatoes + wild mushrooms = **spaghetti bolognese**

TOP TIP 🖉

Research in the *Journal of Sports Medicine* has shown that just 2 minutes of walking within 60–90 minutes of eating a meal can lower blood sugar. Having a lower, more consistent blood sugar leads to more sustained energy. Taking a mini-walk aids digestion and absorption and reduces the likelihood of Type 2 diabetes.

Protecting your nutrients

As well as adding in as many nutrients as possible, it's important to consider how fresh your food is. This has a big impact on the levels of micronutrients. Vegetables can lose anything between 15–77 per cent of their vitamin C content within a week of being picked and, in fact, they start losing their nutrient value as soon as they leave the plant. This is problematic if you're trying to maximize the amount of nutrients in your diet. Nutrient loss is by heat, oxygen and light, so by the time a carrot has languished in your fridge for a few weeks, it's likely that its nutrients will be depleted. Some steps you can take to keep hold of the nutrients in your vegetables are:

- Seek out local farmers' markets, where vegetables might have a shorter lead time between being picked and ending up in your shopping trolley.
- Try to grow your own – even a small window box can produce a lot of salad leaves or herbs.
- Don't cut up your fruit and vegetables until you need to use them, as the protective skin prevents the fruit and vegetables from reacting with oxygen and thus losing antioxidants.
- Don't discount frozen fruit and vegetables as they will have been picked and frozen at their peak nutrient value.
- Try and store vegetables in airtight glass containers in the fridge to enhance shelf life.

Cravings

Be honest, what do you reach for when tiredness strikes? For me, it was always a cookie or chocolate. I remember when I was at my most fatigued I was always looking for a quick fix and for me it was sugar. The confusing thing was it seemed to work – until the crash some hours later when I would either have to take a nap or have another sugary snack. Now, if I eat too much chocolate I feel unwell. I get a headache, feel jittery and need to go to sleep. I find that just having a bit satisfies my cravings without making me feel bad.

The problem with these 'quick fix' coping strategies is that they don't, in fact, help you to cope. The good news is that there are natural substances out there that can act as a pick-me-up without the side effects or dangers of 'traditional' stimulants or drugs. They are less aggressive, more therapeutic solutions for our bodies to encourage greater healing and repair.

If your diet is lacking in nutrients, protein and fibre, you might experience cravings, especially for sugar. This is often because you don't feel sufficiently full. If you find that your weight fluctuates or you struggle with your weight, this could be due to your leptin and ghrelin (the hunger and fullness hormones) being disturbed. Add in poor sleep, which affects the hormones that regulate hunger, fullness and your sleep–wake cycle, plus dehydration and physical inactivity, and you'll further strengthen the crave lifecycle of behaviour. How many processed foods you eat and how often will play a factor. Remember, cravings are your body's way of telling you something isn't right. So, what is your body asking for?

Cravings can be mental as well as physical. Stressful times increase cortisol, which in turn changes eating habits. If you are having a bad day or are in a setting that is associated with a type of food – for example, being at a football match and having a hotdog – that has the same impact. Finally, if you are more of an impulsive person or have an addictive personality, you can be more susceptible to cravings.

The good news is that once you start eating well your taste buds will adapt. Taste bud cells undergo continual turnover even in adulthood, and their average lifespan has been estimated as approximately ten days (Gordon, E. L., et al., 2018). What you never used to enjoy you may start to crave and love. In the meantime, there are some quick fixes you can try if you are prone to cravings:

- taking a chromium supplement, which helps regulate blood sugar levels
- adding cinnamon to food
- having a few tablespoons of lemon or lime juice before, during or after a sugary meal to blunt the glucose spike (Freitas et al., 2020)
- taking some light exercise
- changing your physical space
- eating more regularly to avoid blood sugar dips
- opting for lower GI foods, such as berries, apples,

dark chocolate above 70%, plain yoghurt, chickpeas, peppers and tomatoes
- increasing protein for satiety
- staying hydrated
- making nutrient-dense food swaps, for example swap milk chocolate for nuts (protein) and a few squares of dark chocolate (antioxidants), or crisps for super-thin baked sweet potato (complex carb + antioxidants/ micronutrients) and homemade guacamole, or bread and butter for rye bread or sourdough (complex carb) and nut butter (protein + healthy fats).

TOP TIP ✏️

Gloria Mark from the University of California found that for every disruption, it takes 23 minutes and 15 seconds to get back to full focus after being distracted. By doing something to distract yourself when you're craving poor food choices, you might find yourself able to choose a healthier option.

Nudge theory

Richard Thaler won a Nobel Prize for his research on 'nudging' – the process of making someone make the right choice without using economic incentives.

The research, led by Romain Cardario, found that there are various types of nudge:

Cognitive nudges
Changing someone's mind by trusting the consumer to make the right choice.

Affective nudges
Targeting the heart by making healthy food sound more exciting.

Behavioural nudges
Changing behaviours or persuading consumers to make the right choice.

Supermarkets are a great example of how nudge theory can make customers buy more. Have you ever gone down the aisles, avoided the sugar-laden cereals and cakes and felt proud of yourself for not buying your favourite treats, only to queue up to pay and see delicious chocolate bars displayed nearby at the front of the store? The longer you wait, the harder it gets to resist, and after a while you give in simply because it is right there staring at you, and you have nothing else to do.

So how can you apply the principles of nudge theory to nudge yourself into making the right choices? Here are some examples of enhancements you can make that make doing the right thing easier:

Five Steps to Feeling Less Tired

Convenience enhancements to increase the ease by which consumers make healthy food choices

- Leave fruit and vegetables at the front of the fridge.
- Hide sugary foods or don't have them in the house.
- Leave your gym kit out so it's right in front of you in the morning or wear your gym gear during the day so you can do 5-minute bursts of exercise.
- Have nutritious snacks in your bag at all times.
- Sign up to a regular weekly class.

Size enhancements to either reduce the amount of unhealthy food on the plate or reduce the composition to include more healthy food – 'adding in' nutrients

- Use a different plate to reduce portion size.
- Take small glass/Tupperware boxes out with you filled with nuts and seeds rather than buying a large bag of crisps.
- Opt for a mini 70% dark chocolate bar over a full-sized milk chocolate bar.

Hedonic enhancements to make healthy food more appealing

- Turn typically boring foods, such as quinoa, into something tastier by adding feta, pomegranate seeds and olive oil.
- Take strawberries and dip them in antioxidant-rich dark chocolate.

- Change your normal running route to somewhere new with an amazing view.
- Book in a 'me' day and do whatever you love to do and take some much-needed time out.

THE STAGES OF BEHAVIOUR CHANGE

 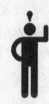

Precontemplation (unaware of the problem)	Contemplation (aware of the problem and of the desired behaviour change)	Preparation (intends to take action)	Action (practises the desired behaviour)	Maintenance (works to sustain the behaviour change)

What about drinks?

Is bottled water better than tap water?

Water is essential for fighting fatigue and the cleaner, the better. Some suggest bottled water tastes better and is superior to tap water, but in many studies where the subjects blind-tasted tap and bottled water, both passed the same taste test (Debbeler et al., 2018).

It may be worth installing a filtering system at your home, but this may not be possible due to budget, space or time constraints. A good filtering system will remove contaminants and improve the overall quality of the water, but a water filter jug is a good cost-effective option. Different filters, similarly to wines, change the taste of the water.

Tap water may contain chemicals such as PFAS (per- and polyfluoroalkyl substances) known as microplastics. Microplastics are endocrine disruptors, and they can cause havoc with our hormones, mimicking oestrogen.

The people most at risk are:

- women who are pregnant or breastfeeding
- those who are immunocompromised
- babies and children

Being dehydrated can have consequences. When 42-year-old Mary came to see me she was very constipated. She complained of feeling sluggish and exhausted and she often couldn't sleep well. She was bloated and had food allergies to wheat, garlic and anything with yeast in it. She was also a yo-yo dieter whose weight had always fluctuated, and when we went through her food and lifestyle diary, I found that she ate a very restricted, bland diet, relying on ready meals, convenience foods and snacks. She drank no water and her only fluid intake was coffee, soft drinks and alcohol. Her urine sample was very dark as she was constantly dehydrated.

When I asked Mary why she didn't drink any water, she said she didn't like the taste, so the focus of her plan was to start hydrating her properly to improve her bloating and gastro-intestinal issues.

First, we added a probiotic to reduce dysbiotic symptoms, added in fibre-rich foods, increased magnesium-rich vegetables, like broccoli and cauliflower, and introduced a magnesium-rich supplement for her constipation. But we really needed to increase her water content. To start with we did this by adding berries such as raspberries to her water, puréed down to make a delicious non-alcoholic Bellini. It worked a treat. In her follow-up she reported that her bowel movements were more regular, her bloating was better and her energy had increased. Her urine was now straw coloured, which showed that she was properly hydrated.

TOP TIP ✏️

Invest in a BPA-free water bottle with a straw. Add lemons or limes, berries, cucumber, apple, fresh mint for 'Pimms' or 'Bellinis' to make the water more palatable. BPA (bisphenol A) has been used to make plastics and resins since the 1950s. Some research has shown that BPA can seep into food or beverages from containers that are made with BPA. It's an endocrine disruptor, meaning it can be neurologically and reproductively toxic.

Coffee

I have a confession to make: I have never actually tried coffee. In fact, I can't bear the smell or taste, even in cakes or ice cream. However, for many people, my family and friends included, a morning latte or flat white is something to look forward to and is crucial for curbing their tiredness. Caffeine is a psychoactive stimulant that increases dopamine and blocks adenosine (which makes us sleepier). When you haven't had a coffee for a while, the adenosine rushes back in, giving you the caffeine crash feeling.

However, some science suggests that coffee can have some health benefits, in particular with performance in sports. Research has shown that those who drink coffee have more diversity in their guts, likely due to the soluble fibre and polyphenol compounds (Gonzalez et al., 2020). The dosage and timing of your daily coffee is what makes it either helpful or harmful. If you want to avoid those coffee crashes, it's advisable to cut down slowly, only consuming as an infrequent rescue remedy and ideally switch to caffeine-free herbal teas or water. Coffee has a half-life of 6–8 hours, meaning that if you drink a coffee at 3 pm, half of it will still will be in your system at 11 pm, which may make it much harder to wind down and sleep. It is advisable to have your last coffee 8–10 hours before you go to sleep. Some people have a genetic sensitivity to caffeine, which makes it more difficult to metabolize it and leaves them feeling wired and tired (Robertson et al., 2018). People with caffeine sensitivity may not be able to metabolize it well in the liver due to a liver enzyme called CYP1A2. If you produce less of this enzyme, you may process and eliminate caffeine from your system more slowly. Signs you may have a caffeine sensitivity are:

- nervousness or anxiousness
- restlessness
- insomnia
- headache
- racing heartbeat

TOP TIP

If you metabolize coffee well, Dr Sarah Myhill suggests adding a teaspoon of D-ribose to organic black coffee. This supports ATP synthesis, resulting in energy production. It's a lifesaving rescue remedy on tired days.

If you'd like to swap coffee for something else, there are some delicious and healthy alternatives:

Dandelion coffee

Research suggests that dandelion coffee is anti-inflammatory, supports blood sugar regulation and has antioxidant properties to neutralize those pesky free radicals. It tastes sweeter and less bitter than standard coffee.

Herbal teas

As with anything, one cup of herbal tea isn't going to turn you from exhausted to energized. But using teas in conjunction with nutrition and other energy-enhancing tools can make a difference. Some herbal teas not only lower cortisol (the stress hormone) but increase the production of mood-enhancing hormones like GABA (gamma-aminobutyric acid) and dopamine. For any herbal tea to be effective, you need to use a therapeutic dose, which is two tea bags as just one often doesn't contain enough of the herb. Keep the pot lid on too to avoid the therapeutic properties of the oils from the tea escaping. Some herbal teas to try and their special naturopathic properties:

- peppermint – bloating, nausea, PMS
- ginger – bloating, sore throat, cold, upset stomach
- green – bloating, allergies, weight loss
- nettle – reduces risk of infection, eye health
- chamomile – sleep, headaches, anxiety, bloating
- matcha – immunity, detoxifier, burns fat

Alcohol

Alcohol is ingrained in our culture. We use it to relax, unwind, be a better version (or so we think) of ourselves, be less inhibited and more confident. The thing is, although alcohol does make us feel these things in the short term, long-term heavy use is a risk factor for fatigue. This is largely due to the fact that it contains toxins, but also because of its sugar content, so choosing lower-sugar alcohol is wise. Here are some sugar contents for different tipples:

Real ale/cider (1 pint) – 9 sugar cubes
Alcopop (700ml bottle) – 7.5 sugar cubes
Vodka and Red Bull (single shot) – 7 sugar cubes
Vodka and Coke (single shot) – 6.5 sugar cubes
Gin and tonic (single shot) – 5.5 sugar cubes
Guinness (1 pint) – 5 sugar cubes
Premium lager (1 pint) – 3.5 sugar cubes
White wine (medium glass) – 2.5 sugar cubes
Baileys (50ml shot) – 2.5 sugar cubes
Rosé wine (medium glass) – 1 sugar cube
Red wine (medium glass) – 0.25 sugar cubes
Prosecco (medium flute) – 0.25 sugar cubes

And, of course, some alcoholic drinks even have health benefits. If you love a glass of Merlot, for example, it's good news as red wine contains antioxidants such as resveratrol, which are said to reduce inflammation and cut the risk of heart disease. However, we still need to remember that cutting back on alcohol can reduce blood pressure, diabetes and heart disease risk, hence why moderation is key. Alcohol works in a similar way to coffee in terms of how well you metabolize it. If you end up with a very red face, for example, this could be a sign that you can't metabolize it well.

The chemistry of a hangover

Hangovers are horrible. They leave you feeling nauseous, shaky and dehydrated and they give you a headache and exhaustion. You either choose fatty, high-carb options to soak it all up or you can't eat due to nausea. Hangovers are like an illness in itself! Or perhaps you are a rare lucky person and don't get hangovers. So why does this actually happen?

It is all to do with something known as acetaldehyde. Alcohol is broken down in our liver by two liver enzymes – ADH and ALDH (alcohol dehydrogenase and aldehyde dehydrogenase if you are interested!). These enzymes break the alcohol down so it can be eliminated out of the body by our urine. ADH helps to convert alcohol into acetaldehyde, which is a very toxic carcinogen. Even though it is only in our bodies for a short period of time, it can cause significant damage to our liver, our pancreas and brains, as sometimes it is metabolized there and in our gastrointestinal tract, which is why alcohol can cause stomach upsets.

Next time you fancy a drink, firstly ask yourself why. Are you bored, stressed, tired or anxious? In which case, is there anything else you could have or do? Secondly, if you do just fancy a drink and, to be clear, there is nothing wrong with this, then choose a high-quality alcohol or opt for a lower alcohol option. If for you the ritual of making a great drink is enjoyable, even some of the no-alcohol options taste superb.

TOP TIP 🖉

Every time we spike our glucose levels by eating a refined sweet food, we are harming our mitochondria. Sugar also disrupts the gut microbiome by promoting the growth of 'bad bacteria', leading to dysbiosis and reducing important immune cells. A tip for every time you want something sweet is to eat something savoury instead.

(https://www.sciencedaily.com/releases/2021/08/210803175250.htm)

Intuitive eating vs emotional eating

You might be thinking: all this is good and well, but it's not that easy to think about the nutritional value of what you eat when you're tired, run down and busy. And you'd be right. On top of that, when we go through hard times, such as a period of stress or even just the cold winters, it's tempting to treat ourselves to foods that don't nourish us. The problem with this is that, when we do, we will feel our energy dip even more. This is because we've created blood sugar dysregulation and our mitochondrial function isn't working as well as it should. Jessie Inchauspe, the Glucose Goddess, talks a lot about blood sugar and says that glucose rollercoasters lead to higher fatigue than diets that flatten glucose curves. By noticing this emotional eating pattern and paying attention to why we're doing it, we can start to turn things around.

Intuitive eating is recognizing what your body needs and when it needs it. The aim is to recognize hunger signals and try to avoid emotional eating. It means stopping before you reach for that sugary snack or takeaway meal and thinking: do I need this? Am I really hungry? It is an important shift in thinking from seeing food as 'good' or 'bad' and enjoying all food as part of a healthy lifestyle.

Weight is an emotive topic. Finding your 'set point' – your natural weight that isn't a struggle to maintain but healthy enough to fuel you throughout the day – can be difficult. What frustrates me most in tackling obesity is the idea that if you struggle with your weight this is because you are overeating and have consumed excess calories. Now this could be true, but obesity could also be due to:

- genetics
- hormonal imbalances, either with the hunger and fullness hormones leptin and ghrelin or a thyroid issue
- not eating the right foods for you and your body
- your gut microbes
- high cortisol levels due to stress

It could even be a combination of all these factors, which is why obesity is complex and can be difficult to treat.

The gentlest and most sustainable way of tackling obesity is by replacing emotional eating with intuitive eating. This might feel like an uphill struggle – or even insurmountable – especially if you've been yo-yo dieting for years. How are you supposed to know how much you need to eat without relying on calorie counting, scales, trackers or portion control?

Here are a few pointers to start you off:

- Identify whether you are physically hungry (a biochemical need) or emotionally hungry (to satisfy a craving or emotion).
- Start simply by including nutrient toppers, micronutrients or antioxidant-rich fruit and vegetables.
- Create the right environment for eating – ideally low stress, relaxed and with a nice atmosphere.
- Eat mindfully, chewing every mouthful.
- It's a marathon not a sprint, so don't hoover your food.
- Don't eat when you feel stressed. Take some time out before you start your meal to unwind first.
- Don't berate yourself for eating 'good' or 'bad' foods, just try and eat nutrient-dense foods most of the time and enjoy your favourite foods in good quality and smaller quantities when you want them.

Of course, when it comes to nutrients and blood sugar, under-eating can be just as problematic as overeating. You might have followed a clean eating, orthorexic or restrictive diet, in which case it is likely you will not be consuming enough. Depriving your body of key macro and micronutrients and cutting out entire food groups is no different to someone who is over-eating energy-dense and nutrient-poor foods. Both are weight disorders but at different ends of the spectrum, and as you are feeding your body too few nutrients, both will lead to poor energy and malnourishment.

The most important thing is to start small. This was the case with Sarah. Aged 56 she was post-menopausal and was struggling with her weight. She felt lethargic, didn't have the energy to exercise and felt demotivated. She was experiencing hot flushes and strong cravings for sugar. When we looked at her diet I could see that it wasn't very diverse. She ate almost the same thing every day: a bagel for breakfast, a sandwich for lunch and something like pasta or a fish pie for dinner. She snacked on chocolate, biscuits and cakes. When we went through her case, it became apparent that she had lost her zest for life. She was divorced, her children had left for university and she wasn't enjoying her career. Because she didn't feel particularly fulfilled and was living on her own, she almost didn't care about what she ate.

This meant she was stuck in a vicious cycle of low energy = low motivation = feeling more unfulfilled. I knew we'd have to start small, so we began by introducing more vegetables and fresh, nutrient-dense foods into her diet. These included broccoli, cabbage and kale. We switched her white rice and white pasta to brown versions to increase fibre content and give her a better blood-sugar balance. Once Sarah had mastered this habit, we slowly encouraged her to switch the snacks for lower-sugar, higher-nutrient varieties. We discussed options together and chose things she loved the sound of, such as roasted chickpeas with paprika, Greek yoghurt, berries and nut butter and banana muffins made without refined sugar. Slowly she started to feel more energized. And because she did, she joined a group exercise class where she met some lovely people. By tackling her diet first and making tiny changes, Sarah had enough energy to start reviewing other areas of her life. At her follow-up, Sarah said she felt like a different person and is still continuing to follow a much healthier lifestyle and using the power of community to keep her going.

TOP TIP 🖊

Eating late increases hunger, decreases calories burned and changes fat tissue that may increase obesity risk, proving that it isn't just what we eat, but when we eat too (Brigham and Women's Hospital, 2022). Trying to eat at the same times every day and stopping eating your last meal at 7.30 pm will not only improve your sleep, but also research shows having a longer eating window between your dinner and eating your breakfast the next day can help with weight loss. I do believe in leaving a minimum of a 12–14-hour window between dinner and breakfast, i.e. 8 pm to 8 am or 7.30 pm to 9.30 am.

TOP TIP

Don't try to overhaul your whole diet at once. Start small, making a couple of meaningful swaps, such as brown rice instead of white, an extra portion of vegetables you don't normally eat or include a protein source with every meal and snack.

Following a BIG way of eating isn't about denying yourself or cutting out what you like. In fact, it should start by adding in nutrient-dense delicious food to what you already eat. It's time to let go of the idea that healthy eating revolves around dieting, punishment and deprivation. Instead, start building your plate in a way that feels balanced for you, using colour, being as diverse as you can and including some nutrient toppers as a way of adding in additional micronutrients. Learning how to be consistent and not getting into a cycle of feast and famine will allow your body to maintain its weight and, more importantly, give your cells a consistent flow of energy.

KEY ACTIONS IN STEP 1: FUEL YOUR BODY

- BIG nutrition is about supporting your Brain, Immune system and Gut through adding nutritionally dense foods into your diet, not taking away.
- Use this formula to build each plate of food you eat: **Protein + healthy fats + complex carbs + antioxidants and micronutrients**.
- The top three most nutritionally dense foods in the world are salmon, kale and seaweed.
- Add nutrient toppers to food to increase your micronutrients. Try seeds, nori flakes, tree nuts or coconut flakes.
- Berries, leafy greens and egg yolks are all rich in tryptophan, which work more effectively when combined with 25–30 grams of carbohydrates.

Step 2

Support Your Gut
Energy from the inside out

The microbe is nothing. The terrain is everything.

Louis Pasteur

Do you ever get that sinking or lurching feeling in your stomach when something doesn't feel quite right? It might be a decision you're about to make, or a job or relationship you find yourself in, or it might be for no particular reason at all. We call it our 'gut instinct'. But why does it come from the gut?

I had this exact feeling some years ago when I was about to launch a new wellness business. I'd worked tirelessly to set up the venture, but just at the point of launch I felt this sense of gnawing in my stomach. It wasn't fear, it was just a sense of uneasiness that I couldn't shift. I kept waking up in the middle of the night and, despite knowing that everything was fine in my brain, I had these strange sensations in my gut. Despite all the work, expense and time I'd spent building the business, I decided to pause the launch so I could reflect on why I was having these feelings. After some time, I realized that I was being driven solely by money and my ego and I wasn't even the right person to run this type of business. It would require a strong logistics and supply chain background, neither of which I had experience in or had any desire to manage.

After a lot of soul-searching, I pulled the plug on the whole thing. Eventually, I built and launched my nutrition clinic and platform, NOCO Health, which supports people with energy issues and burnout. It's a smaller business but one I am hugely passionate about.

Why did I get that feeling in my gut and not my brain? What's so special about our digestive system that it seems to be able to communicate? Well, it turns out that while your head and your heart can lie to you, your gut never does.

The gut contains millions of neurons not that different to the ones in your brain. In fact, the gut and the brain are intrinsically linked, and even communicate with each other via the vagus nerve, the longest nerve in the autonomic nervous system. This is why we get butterflies in our tummy when we're nervous or can get an upset stomach in times of stress. It's why many of our deep feelings seem to come from the gut. Because, just like your brain, your gut is desperately trying to send you messages all the time. But how often do we listen?

The gut is known as the 'second brain' because its diverse bacteria help produce neurotransmitters such as serotonin, nor-epinephrine, dopamine, GABA, acetylcholine and melatonin, all of which control our feelings and emotions and affect cognition. This is why it is not only important to listen to your gut, but to nourish it correctly too. The gut tract mucosa is the largest surface between us and the outside world and is where most diseases occur.

The primary functions of the gut microbiome are to:

- break down fibre
- synthesize vitamins
- produce neurotransmitters
- stimulate the immune system
- fight off pathogenic microbes to help prevent inflammation and allergies
- genetic expression
- appetite regulation
- blood sugar regulation
- produces food for the mitochondria, which is how we generate energy in our cells
- detoxification, such as hormones

GUT HEALTH: ENERGY FROM THE INSIDE OUT

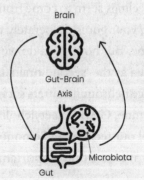

Brain

Influence on:
motility secretion
nutrient delivery
microbial balance

Gut-Brain
Axis

Influence on:
neurotransmitters
stress/anxiety
mood
behaviour

Microbiota

Gut

Rebooting your gut

In Step 1 we started to improve nutrition by adding nutrient-rich foods to your diet. This will be an ongoing process and one you can gradually increase as you make more small changes to what you eat. The next step is to tackle the microbiome of your gut – in other words, the balance of bacteria that keeps everything working as it should. Restoring and supporting intestinal health and the integrity of the gut barrier are two of the most important things that you can do. Gut dysbiosis – an imbalance of these bacteria – can be a significant factor not only in the symptoms of fatigue but in acne, anxiety, auto-immune conditions, brain fog, joint and muscle pain, chronic headaches, migraines and more. Since your digestive tract is where most of your immune cells are and where you absorb your nutrients, it makes sense that improving gut health can improve your health across your whole body. In this chapter we're going to start to correct gut dysbiosis by 'rebooting your gut'. We're going to:

- Cleanse
- Populate
- Heal
- Maintain

So, what's involved?

Cleanse

First, we want to remove anything that could be irritating the gut. This could include:

Trigger foods

These include any type of gut irritant, such as alcohol, caffeine, processed food and food additives. You might have a hard time digesting certain types of carbohydrates, like bread or pasta, or you might have a food intolerance, sensitivity or food allergy. By removing the likely culprits one at a time, we can find out what these are.

Medications and supplements

Over-the-counter medications, such as heartburn medication and NSAIDs (like aspirin and ibuprofen), are known to cause digestive dysfunction, as are many prescription medications. Many supplements can cause digestive symptoms, so at this stage we want to remove anything you do not need to take. A nutritionist can support your goal of coming off any prescription medication, but it has to be done with the full support of your doctor and under supervision.

Stress

The hypothalamus releases a hormone called CRH, or corticotropin-releasing hormone. CRH signals to the pituitary gland to secrete ACTH, or adrenocorticotropin hormone, into the bloodstream. It travels into the adrenal glands where it prompts the release of cortisol, which causes the changes that help the body deal with stress. Stress isn't just a feeling. It causes a biochemical reaction by releasing a hormone called cortisol into your bloodstream, and too much cortisol can cause inflammation in the digestive tract. Removing stress from your life is easier said than done, but at this stage we want to try to reduce it as much as possible. The easiest and quickest way to do this is by simplifying your life, even if just for a short period. That might mean taking some time off work, mending some tricky relationships or asking for help with the cooking or cleaning for a few weeks.

Infections, bacteria, parasites and pathogens

Now is the time to have some stool tests to check you don't have any bugs that might require treatment. Your doctor will offer a basic stool test and there are plenty of companies that offer a more comprehensive test. However, these can be expensive and difficult to interpret without an expert walking you through your results, so I advise you trying to reboot your gut first, especially if your symptoms are mild.

Toxins

Toxins are all around us and difficult to escape completely, but there's a lot you can do to reduce your exposure. Take another look at the questionnaire in Chapter 5 (see page 95) to assess your personal exposure to toxins. If you came out as medium or high risk, don't panic – you can reduce your exposure significantly by:

Five Steps to Feeling Less Tired

- Changing your regular cleaning and toiletry products to a non-toxic brand.
- Using an app such as Yuka or Think Dirty to find out about potentially toxic ingredients in your foods, cosmetics and personal care products and making switches accordingly.
- Changing exercise routes to less polluted areas.
- Storing foods in glass jars and cooking with stainless steel not aluminium pans.
- Getting a mould specialist to come and check your home and reduce mould exposure. Your local council may do this for free.
- Forgoing makeup by embracing the natural look, using chemical-free makeup and toiletries or wearing your normal makeup brands less often.
- Switching your sun cream to one that is chemical free.
- Buying organic for the 'dirty dozen' – the foods that are most likely to be contaminated with toxins. These are strawberries, spinach, kale, apples, nectarines, grapes, peppers, cherries, peaches, pears, celery and tomatoes. There are also 'the clean 15', which are the fruit and vegetables least likely to be contaminated. They are avocados, sweetcorn, pineapple, onions, papaya, sweet peas (frozen), asparagus, honeydew melon, kiwi,

cabbage, mushrooms, cantaloupe melon,
mangoes, watermelon and sweet potatoes.

Last year, the American Environmental Working Group (EWG) analyzed 500 leading sunscreen products. They discovered they could only recommend 39 of them. Some research suggests these products are actually causing skin cancer rather than preventing it. There appears to be two primary ingredients to avoid:

Vitamin A derivative known as retinyl palmitate
This may have photocarcinogenic properties, which can rapidly increase cancer formation with sun exposure.

Free radicals
Many sunscreens have free radical-generating properties called benzophenones, which block the UVA and UVB light that damages the skin. However, these disrupt enzyme production and can go into the blood via the skin, damaging cells.

Over the page are some other 'Red List' ingredients to avoid with common toiletry products:

Five Steps to Feeling Less Tired

RED LIST

Shampoo

✗ Ethanolamines
(cocamide DEA and others)
✗ Parabens (e.g. butylparabens)
✗ UV filters (Octinoxate, Oxybenzone)
✗ Formaldehyde-releasing
preservatives (diazolidinyl urea,
imidazolidinyl urea, DMDM hydantoin)
✗ Sodium Laureth Sulfate and other -eth
compounds, which can be contaminated
with 1.4-dioxane and ethylene oxide

Conditioner

✗ Ethanolamines
(cocamide DEA and others)
✗ Parabens (e.g. butylparaben)
✗ Formaldehyde-releasing preservatives
(diazolidinyl urea, imidazolidinyl urea,
DMDM hydantoin)
✗ Sodium Laureth Sulfate and other -eth
compounds, which can be contaminated
with 1.4-dioxane and ethylene oxide
✗ Hydrogenated cottonseed oil, which
can be contaminated with arsenic
✗ Nonoxynols, which can be contaminated
with 1.4-dioxane and ethylene oxide

Moisturizer/ Anti-Ageing Creams

✗ Polyacrylamide,
acrylamide contamination
✗ PTFE, PFOA contamination
✗ Placental extracts (can contain
progesterone or estrogen)
✗ UV filters (octinoxate,
oxybenzone, homosalate)
✗ Petroleum, PAH contamination

Sunscreen

✗ Benzophenone
✗ Homosalate
✗ Octinoxate
✗ Oxybenzone
✗ Padimate O
✗ Para-aminobenzoic acid (PABA)

Blush, Eye Shadow & Face Powders

✗ Titanium dioxide
✗ Carbon black
✗ PTFE
✗ Talc
✗ BHA
✗ Silica
✗ Formaldehyde-releasing preservatives
(quaternium-15, imidazolidinyl urea)

Hair Colour

✗ Resorcinol
✗ p-Phenylenediamine
✗ Toluene
✗ Lead acetate
✗ Ethanolamines
(cocamide DEA and others)

Populate

Elimination diets are not forever, and it's important not to cut out food groups for long as the gut needs a variety of foods for it to work well. Once symptoms have improved significantly, it's time to reintroduce foods and supplements that will help rebalance the microbiome – your collection of good gut bacteria that play a role in immune, digestive and metabolic health. These are called probiotics and prebiotics.

Research suggests that probiotics:

Aid the body in absorbing key nutrients
When the body has too few beneficial bacteria or too many pathogenic strains, this can impact the absorption of key nutrients from your food.

Improve the quality and quantity of your sleep
Supplementing with probiotics can reduce cortisol production and taking probiotics can boost tryptophan production in the body. The gut is largely responsible for the production of serotonin and melatonin, both hormones important for sleep. Serotonin, our happy hormone, is vital for maintaining melatonin levels and regulating a healthy sleep cycle.

Improve blood sugar levels
The Lactobacillus reuteri strain helps achieve optimal insulin and glucose levels.

Foods rich in probiotics include:

- yoghurt
- sauerkraut
- kimchi
- pickled vegetables
- kombucha
- kefir

You'll see that these are all fermented foods. Fermented foods contain GABA, a neurotransmitter that blocks signals to the brain. Now, you may think that doesn't sound good, but GABA has an inhibitory effect when it attaches to a protein called the GABA receptor and actually calms the nervous system, reducing stress and anxiety.

If these don't sound that enticing then remember you can add them into your diet in the form of a 'topper' to your stir-fries, salads, veggies or rice. You can also buy kefir yoghurt, which you can substitute for normal yoghurt.

TOP TIP 🖉

Try to have one 'shot' of fermented foods
every day, either as a side accompaniment or
mix them into your rice or veg. This is more
effective than consuming a large quantity
irregularly.

Eating more plants is a great way of introducing more gut diversity because plants have a microbiome too. It's known as the rhizosphere environment – the important soil zone where all the amazing minerals can be found. The rhizosphere isn't just important for the health of the plant, but for our gut health, too. The Human Microbiome project, a gargantuan study about the gut microbiome carried out between 2007 and 2016, started to piece together the connection between the quality of the soil microbiome and that of our guts. It discovered that microbes contribute more of the genes responsible for our survival than the genes we were born with. It found that our health depends not only on our own microbes but on the microbes we ingest from the soil – either directly from the dirt we get on our hands or indirectly from the plants that we eat.

However, it's fair to say that the rhizosphere isn't what it once was. Due to intensive farming methods and pesticides, there is a lack of biodiversity in our soil and because of this compromised soil quality, our gut microbiomes aren't as diverse either. The message is that it's important where and how your plant foods were grown. Again, growing your own would be the best option here, especially as you will get dirt on your hands! If that's not possible, the next best thing is to have an understanding of how the vegetables you buy are grown and the quality of the soil they've come from. Buying locally and seasonally should help with this, so seek out your local markets, greengrocers and farm shops and ask them questions.

As well as eating some of the foods mentioned and getting your hands dirty, you can also buy probiotics as a supplement.

However, the sheer number of different types available make choosing the right probiotic a minefield. How do you know what to buy?

You might be tempted to buy the probiotic that has the highest number of strains, for example 5 billion. But more doesn't necessarily mean better. What's more important is that you take the best probiotic strains for your symptoms. Here are some common probiotic strains and the symptoms they support:

Bifidobacterium
- supports digestion
- helps reduce infection
- prevents catching flu and colds
- improves lactose digestion
- supports respiratory and heart health

Lactobacillus
- supports healthy weight management
- reduces UTI and yeast infections
- supports digestion
- prevents catching flu and colds

L. plantarum
- aids abdominal discomfort
- reduces gas and bloating
- promotes bowel regularity

You can also find these probiotic strains in things like kimchi, sauerkraut, yoghurt, cheese and cultured vegetables.

In addition to probiotics, our gut needs prebiotics. These feed the good bacteria in the gut. They then produce useful nutrients like short-chain fatty acids, such as butyrate, acetate or propionate and contribute to protection from infection and inflammation (Fukuda et al., 2011), which keep the intestines working. Prebiotic foods include:

- apples
- apple cider vinegar
- asparagus
- bananas
- barley
- berries
- chicory
- cocoa
- flaxseed
- raw garlic
- green vegetables
- Jerusalem artichokes
- leeks
- legumes (peas and beans)
- oats
- onions
- tomatoes

Heal

Next, we want to create an environment that provides long-term support for the gut, so we need to repair the intestinal cells and mucosa and reduce inflammation. This might include introducing:

- Foods high in vitamins A, C, D and E, as well as the mineral zinc (see pages 180–83 for a list of these).
- Foods rich in amino acids, such as bone broth.
- Supplements such as L-glutamine, collagen, aloe vera, marshmallow or slippery elm.

If you're suffering with tiredness and/or other symptoms, you might be lacking stomach acid, bile and digestive enzymes. You can increase these by including:

- Foods containing nutrients that help the body produce these elements. For instance, bitter foods such as bitter melon or cruciferous vegetables like kale and cabbage can help stimulate stomach acid and digestive enzymes. You can buy a herbal bitters complex.
- Foods and/or supplements to address nutrient deficiencies. Digestive conditions can affect the absorption of nutrients such as B12, iron, calcium, magnesium and zinc. This can be common with those following a vegan or vegetarian diet. See

pages 181 and 183 for a list of foods that are high in these micronutrients.

- Supplements to replace the missing elements such as betaine HCL, bile salts and enzymes. You can include natural digestive enzymes – papain and bromelain, which come from papaya and pineapple that help to break down food and improve absorption.
- Other foods high in digestive enzymes include raw miso paste, apple cider vinegar, bee pollen, kiwi fruit, mango, raw honey, sauerkraut and kimchi, kefir and yoghurt and avocados.

Maintain

Our lifestyle habits have an enormous influence on our digestive system and health, so it's vital that once we've rebooted the gut we take long-term steps to maintain a healthy microbiome. During this phase, we want to address:

- stress management techniques to support us through life's inevitable stressful periods
- improved sleep and, more importantly, overall sleep quality
- increased movement (or decreased if over-exercising is a problem)

We'll cover each of these in the next steps.

Diversify your gut microbiome

Groundbreaking research provides us with an alternative view-point to the five-a-day approach. The optimal number of plants according to *The American Gut Microbiome Study* is 30. In this study, they found those who consumed 30 plants a week had more diverse gut microbes, leading to much better health outcomes than those that consumed less than 10 plants.

This may sound a lot, but this includes pulses and legumes, nuts and seeds, wholegrains, fruits and vegetables and herbs and spices.

Switch counting calories to counting plant points.

30 PLANT POINTS A WEEK - WHAT COUNTS?

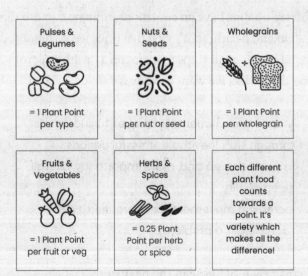

Pulses & Legumes	Nuts & Seeds	Wholegrains
= 1 Plant Point per type	= 1 Plant Point per nut or seed	= 1 Plant Point per wholegrain

Fruits & Vegetables	Herbs & Spices	Each different plant food counts towards a point. It's variety which makes all the difference!
= 1 Plant Point per fruit or veg	= 0.25 Plant Point per herb or spice	

3 simple tips to increase plant diversity in your meals:

- Half the meat in your spaghetti bolognese and add lentils instead.
- Instead of buying an iceberg lettuce, buy mixed leaves – very quickly you go from 1 to potentially 7 points.
- Add frozen vegetables like cauliflower or spinach to smoothies.

KEY ACTIONS FOR STEP 2: SUPPORT YOUR GUT

- Follow the Cleanse, Populate, Heal, Maintain protocol to reboot the gut and rebalance the microbiome.
- Cleanse the gut of trigger foods, toxins, unnecessary medications and supplements.
- Populate the gut with good bacteria from probiotics and feed that bacteria with prebiotics.
- Heal the gut by introducing digestive enzymes and foods rich in amino acids.
- Maintain a healthy gut by reducing stress, improving sleep and regulating movement.

Step 3

Supercharge Your Sleep and Exercise *Balancing movement and rest*

When my CFS was at its worst, I actually struggled to stay awake. If I saw friends, I would have to leave after a few hours because I'd eat and then want to fall asleep straight afterwards. I was known for going to parties and being asleep on the sofa, which looking back now seems so strange. I certainly wasn't the life and soul of the party! The problem was, no matter how much I slept, I never felt refreshed.

I found exercise exhausting. I knew moving my body would be good for me and give me energy, but it became a vicious cycle: the more I moved, the more tired I would become.

In this step, we're going to look at everything you can do to optimize sleep and movement so your mitochondria can heal and start producing a steady flow of energy again. Both rest and exercise are vital in your recovery but managing them can be a difficult tightrope to walk.

Building a sleep routine

To begin, we'll gain a basic understanding of what happens to us when we are sleeping. There are four phases to one night of sleep. N1 is the hazy stage where we drift into the land of sleep. It can last anywhere from 1–5 minutes. Next is the N2 phase. This is where your brain activity, your heart rate and your respiratory rate slows down and can last from 10–60 minutes. Then we reach N3, which is the deep sleep phase, critical for restoring your body and mind. This part is filled with delta waves that help to process your memories and activities from the day and this is when growth hormones are released to repair muscles, bone cells and strengthen the immune system. Lastly, we reach N4, or what is more commonly known as the Rapid Eye Movement (REM) stage, where your brain is almost as active as it is when you're awake. It is when you'll have the most vivid dreams, and these dreams often work to clean out unnecessary information. These phases repeat themselves throughout the night, sometimes five or six times. (https://www.sleepfoundation.org/stages-of-sleep).

We are all biochemically unique so the amount of sleep we need will vary from person to person, but the science suggests that aiming for 8.4 hours is a good start if you want to achieve high energy levels (Sanz Milone et al., 2021). You might think sleep is all about the amount you're getting, but while sleep duration is important, it's only one factor in what makes a good night's sleep. What you might not know is that good sleep starts as soon as you wake up. The amount of light exposure you get in the day, what you eat and how much you move all affect your night's sleep. But why?

The two most important factors in how our body sleeps are the circadian rhythm and what's known as the homeostatic sleep drive. The circadian rhythm is our internal schedule, which determines when we sleep and when we wake. It's driven by many factors, including our chronotype, how much daylight we get, when we eat our meals and when and how much we exercise. Regulating the circadian rhythm is vital when setting a good sleep routine.

Homeostatic sleep drive is the pressure to sleep – in other words, how 'hungry' we are for sleep as the day goes on. Sleep debt is when your sleep quality is less than your body needs across a period of at least two weeks.

Optimizing our circadian rhythm and sleep drive to avoid a sleep debt is critical. To do it, we need to look at our whole day.

First thing in the morning

As soon as you wake up, try to get some natural light, ideally outside as artificial light or sunlight through a window doesn't have the same effect as direct sunlight. Aim for a minimum of 30 minutes within an hour of waking. Getting natural light in the early part of the day regulates everything from melatonin production to cortisol levels and teaches your body when to wake and when to sleep.

Mid-morning

If you want to consume sugar or caffeine, try to do this earlier in the day to avoid high blood sugar levels before bed. Avoid caffeine after lunch. Aim to exercise earlier in the day to avoid a spike in endorphins just before bed.

Halfway through the day

If you are very tired and need to nap, try to do this equidistant between the time you wake up and the time you go to bed. So, if you wake up at 7 am and go to bed at 11 pm, take a nap at around 3 pm.

Just before bedtime

Eat two kiwis before bed. Kiwis contain serotonin, which regulates the sleep cycle (St Onge, 2016). You could also try taking a supplement that includes Montmorency cherries. Studies suggest that due to their high levels of tryptophan and melatonin, cherries induce longer and better-quality sleep. Magnesium is another sleep inducer. Add two cups of magnesium flakes to a bath or take a magnesium-rich supplement, such as magnesium glycinate. This contains glycine, which can reduce anxiety.

You could try doing something that challenges your brain before bed. Research shows that doing something cognitively difficult can allow you to fall asleep more quickly because it increases the homeostatic sleep drive. Puzzles aid relaxation and may reduce stress and anxiety, creating a more optimal sleep environment for your mind and body. Learning a language before bed is a way to get yourself to sleep and studies show you are more likely to remember the new words and phrases if you sleep soon after learning them.

Reading before you sleep could relax you significantly. Cognitive Neuropsychologist Dr David Lewis found that 'Reading worked best, reducing stress levels by 68 per cent.' It was better than listening to music (61 per cent), drinking tea or coffee (54 per cent) and taking a walk (42 per cent). It only took 6 minutes for participants' stress levels to be reduced.

When Fran came to see me she was having trouble sleeping and her energy levels were low. She naturally woke early, which suited her as she had a baby and a full-time job. Fran loved to exercise, but the only time she could fit this in was in the evenings once her baby had gone to bed. She liked to push herself to the limit and immediately after exercising she would feel great. However, she then found it increasingly difficult to go to sleep and would wake the next morning exhausted.

We worked out that by exercising late in the evening, Fran was inadvertently increasing her cortisol levels. By pushing herself hard, she was increasing her core body temperature and releasing endorphins, which, although they made her feel great, were not allowing her to get into a sleep-like state. Fran was clearly a morning chronotype but due to her circumstances was acting as an evening chronotype. Over the course of a few weeks, we made some adjustments to her eating patterns and moved her exercise schedule to include an early-morning run outside in the daylight before work. Although it was tough for a while, after a few weeks Fran's sleep and energy levels were back to normal.

To nap or not to nap

Just as our circadian rhythm plays a vital role in how well we sleep, so does our homeostatic sleep drive. If you have CFS, this appetite for sleep might feel very strong. When this is the case, it's tempting to spend a lot of time in bed, but sleeping late, staying in bed during the day or taking a nap in the afternoon all disturb night-time sleep by weakening the homeostatic sleep drive.

HOMEOSTATIC SLEEP DRIVE IS THE PRESSURE TO SLEEP

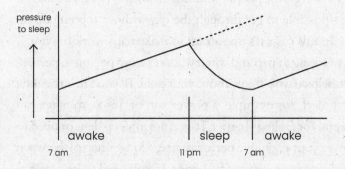

(cdc.gov)

As you can see from this chart, your sleep drive naturally builds throughout your time awake, then tails off as you sleep and increases again when you wake up. When the drive is interrupted – for example, by sleeping during the day – the quality and quantity of your night-time sleep is reduced.

Conversely, several factors can increase the sleep drive:

- A compromised immune system. The more immune cytokines we produce to fight infection, the more our sleep drive increases. This is why we sleep more when we are ill.
- Cognitive exertion, e.g. thinking about something challenging.
- Increased physical exertion.

Ideally, when setting a new sleep routine you would cut out naps entirely to increase this 'sleep appetite' when it's time to go to bed. However, for people suffering from severe fatigue it's not always possible to get through the day without topping up on sleep. In this case, it's important to make naps work for you.

How long to nap and when will vary from person to person, but it helps if you think about your goal. If you are struggling to stay alert, for example, a power nap of 10–20 minutes can be useful for feeling sharper. If you are in sleep debt or need to improve your cognitive performance, a longer nap of between 40 and 90 minutes might be better. If you need to be creative, a nap of 60 minutes or more will ensure you settle into rapid eye movement sleep (REM). The only consideration with this is 'sleepability': how easy someone finds it to nap. Some people find it much easier than others to fall asleep on demand (Harrison and Horne, 1996).

As we discussed above, the timing of your nap is important. While this depends largely on your unique chronotype and how much of a sleep debt you are in, as a general rule it's best to avoid having a nap too late in the day, otherwise you will struggle to fall asleep at night.

NAP TIPS

- Set an alarm to avoid overdosing on sleep, known as sleep inertia.
- Create the right environment to optimize the time.
- Turn off your worries for the duration by doing a short meditation for 5 minutes beforehand.

Knowing when to rest

Sometimes just knowing when to rest and be kind to yourself on low-energy days is crucial to regaining your energy. Christine Miserandino's Spoon Theory uses spoons to depict a unit of energy or a task.

ONE SPOON = ONE TASK

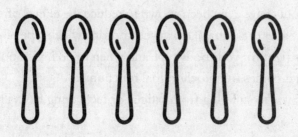

Miserandino suffered with lupus and felt chronically tired. Using the spoons for tasks, she could show how easy it was to use up precious energy. Each spoon represented a task, such as making her bed, cooking a meal or seeing a friend, and it very quickly showed her friend starting with 12 spoons, how easy it is to burn through energy reserves.

Use this theory to consider how much energy you are actually burning through each day and build in proper rest breaks. How many tasks are you doing a day and do you have enough spoons to complete them? Are all of them a priority or can some of them wait for another day? It is a simple concept, but one that will allow you to give your energy to the right tasks as you have a limited number of spoons. What can wait, what can you delegate and what task can you ask for help with?

Managing exercise

Movement is vital for glucose regulation, and both resistance training and aerobic exercise help to maintain a steady blood sugar. Exercise is key in mitochondrial function, and HIIT workouts have even been shown to reduce the effects of sleep debt (Saner et al., 2021). However, knowing which type of exercise is right for your body type and when to do it is important when it comes to mitochondrial function.

If you're suffering from fatigue or recovering from illness, it's even more important to moderate exercise to protect your mitochondria. We've been given a mentality that we have to work out for extended periods, but for many people with fatigue that doesn't work. By making exercise accessible and committing to only working out for ten minutes a day, it will feel restorative rather than a chore.

If you are sitting on the sofa feeling exhausted and you are so tired that a very tiny walk would make your symptoms worse, then don't do it. However, if your brain is tired but your body feels OK, try and get out and see how your body feels. Go easy and be kind to yourself. The fresh air and gentle movement may just start off that protein production for our mitochondria and give you that much-needed energy boost. If you can't muster up a walk, consider sitting or lying down outside if it's sunny.

Ideally, our bodies need aerobic exercise + strength training to keep our energy levels up, as while aerobic exercise increases mito function, resistance training increases the number of mitochondria you have. The more mitos there are, the less chance they'll end up overworked. When we are fatigued this could look like:

Walking (aerobic) + yoga (strength)
Gentle bike ride (aerobic) + Pilates (strength)
Swimming (aerobic) + resistance training (strength)

Pace/nutrient ratio

If you are feeling low in energy, consider your pace/nutrient ratio.

If you are over-pacing (expending too much energy through work or exercise) and under-nourishing, by not consuming enough nutrient-rich food, this can lead to an energy deficit. To close the gap, you can:

- Reduce your pace. Slow down, take rest breaks and find ways to relax.
- Increase your intake of nutrient-rich foods. Focus on those that support the energy-production process (salmon, tuna, brown rice, eggs, etc.), and reduce those that hinder it, such as junk food and sugar, which are not naturally occurring fuels.

In the short term, reduce your pace as a quick fix.

In the longer term, look to increase nutrient-dense foods in your daily diet. This will make the biggest difference to your energy.

THE 5-4-3-2-1 WORKOUT

5 minutes

- any cardio you want, walk, run, elliptical, bike
  If you're at home:
  - 1 min high knees
  - 1 min jumping jacks
  - 1 min front kicks
  - 1 min jumping jacks
  - 1 min run in place

4 minutes

- 1 min lunges or walking lunges
  - 1 min mountain climbers
  - repeat for 4 minutes

3 minutes

- 10 push-ups/rest
- 15 tricep dips/rest
- repeat for 3 minutes

2 minutes

- 30 seconds regular squats
- 30 seconds jump squats
- 30 seconds regular squats
- 30 seconds jump squats

1 minute

- plank

total time 15 mins; intermediate: repeat for 2x through; advanced: repeat for 3x through

- drink H_2O + take breaks whenever you need them

(Source: Printable 5-4-3-2-1 Home Workout)

KEY ACTIONS IN STEP 3: SUPERCHARGE YOUR SLEEP AND EXERCISE

- The key ingredients for sleep are your circadian rhythm and your sleep drive.
- Maximize natural light early in the day to set your circadian rhythm and avoid caffeine and exercise later in the afternoon.
- If you have to nap, do so halfway between waking and going to bed.
- Aerobic exercise and strength training are vital for mitochondrial function.
- Consider adjusting your pace/nutrient ratio to reduce your energy gap.

Step 4

Energize with Supplements
Why, what and when

We've seen how BIG nutrition, gut health, sleep and exercise are the first steps to fixing long-term fatigue. The next step is to look at additional ways we can help our body – and our mitochondria – to start producing enough energy again. Although they will never replace good nutrition, sleep and movement, there are many times when supplements will be the answer to giving your body the boost it needs.

You should consider taking supplements if:

- you have been ill, e.g. with a virus
- you've felt very tired for a long time despite changing your diet
- you are vegan or vegetarian
- you have an illness, such as anaemia
- you are pregnant or breastfeeding
- you suffer with gastrointestinal issues
- you are over 60

You could consider supplementation if you experience any of the following symptoms alongside your fatigue, as they might be a sign of a specific vitamin or mineral deficiency:

- eyelid twitching is a sign of magnesium deficiency
- restless legs
- pins and needles
- cracks in the sides of the mouth (stomatitis)
- mouth ulcers
- brittle hair and nails
- scaly patches or dandruff
- red or white bumps on the skin, such as behind the arms (keratosis pilaris)

Even if you're not experiencing any of these symptoms, there could be a place for supplements in your diet. As we discussed in Step 2 (see page 155), our soil's microbiome is not as diverse as it once was. It's not as rich in vitamins and minerals as it used to be, due to pesticides and intensive farming. This means that the nutrient-status of plant foods is less than it was a few decades ago. Add in modern processing methods, storage and transportation, and the result is that a lot of the nutrients in our food are lost.

As a result, even if we think we are eating a healthy diet and including as many different micronutrients as we can, we will often still struggle to get enough nutrients from the food we eat. In some cases, we would need to consume more than is physically possible just to reach the RDA. This is where supplements come in.

Finding the one that you need

Supplements are a great way to boost your micronutrient levels at particular times. However, there are times when supplements can do more harm than good. Many products are poor quality and contain ingredients we shouldn't be consuming, such as fillers and binders known as excipients. Here are a few ingredients to watch out for when choosing supplements:

- magnesium silicate – can cause health issues when digested
- magnesium stearate – a binder that might be unsafe for humans to consume
- titanium dioxide – a colourant linked to some cancers
- carrageenan – a thickening agent that can inflame the digestive tract
- potassium sorbate – a preservative that can cause allergies

How to select a supplement:

- Always buy from a reputable healthcare source. Many supplements can be counterfeit or low quality from large online retailers.

- Make sure you know why you are taking it. Do you have a deficiency or particular need? If not, don't take supplements just for the sake of it. Have some blood tests first.
- If you have any questions, ask to speak to the supplements clinical team from the company that you buy the supplement from and make sure you are selecting the right product for your needs.
- Register with the supplement companies' websites and take advantage of their promotions and bulk buy to save money.

What to take and when

If you find the world of supplements confusing and expensive, you're not alone. How are you supposed to know what to take, why, what and when? And how much? First things first, if you are currently taking any medication, it's important that you check with your doctor or nutrition practitioner before you start any supplements, as many of the most commonly prescribed medications negatively interact with supplements and herbs.

The dosage really does depend on how severe the issue is and whether you are working with a qualified practitioner. If you are, they may suggest taking a UL dose – the tolerable upper intake level – which is the maximum you can take without any serious side effects. However, if you aren't working with a nutritionist, it is best to stick to the dose suggested on the bottle.

Next, you need to understand which supplements to take for the symptoms you're experiencing. Of course, all vitamins and minerals are important within the body. However, some are more important than others when it comes to energy production and reducing fatigue.

Absorption

Sometimes when we have low energy, it could be because even though we are eating a seemingly nutritious diet and taking supplements, we have an issue with absorption. Antibiotics, lactose intolerance, damage to the intestine where absorption takes place from infection or inflammation, low stomach acid, reduced digestive enzymes so our food cannot be broken down properly or to the simple fact that we're not taking the supplements correctly can all affect absorption.

Two ways of improving absorption are to combine certain vitamins and minerals and take them at the right time of the day and chew more mindfully. Many of these micronutrients work synergistically together and one without the other will have a hard time getting to where it needs to get to within your body. Here are some common supplement pairings, advice on when to take them and what could be hindering absorption:

WATER SOLUBLE VITAMINS

Vitamin/mineral	Best absorption	What helps	What hinders	Deficiency	Food source	Function
B1 Thiamine	Alone or with meals	B complex, manganese	Stress, antibiotics, alcohol	Impaired nervous function and energy production Affects skin and digestive tract, loss of appetite, fatigue	Meat, fish, poultry, eggs, flaxseeds, tahini, beans, pulses	Energy production Helps cells convert food into energy critical for nerve function Protein metabolism
B2 Riboflavin	Alone or with meals	B complex	Nicotine, stress, antibiotics, alcohol	Sores on lips and cracks – cheilosis (cheilitis), dermatitis/eczema Eye problems – itching, blurred vision, sensitivity to light	Meat, fish, eggs, nuts, seeds, green leafy vegetables	Energy production Carbohydrate, fat and protein metabolism Tissue maintenance. Growth and reproduction
B3 Niacin	Alone or with meals	B complex	Stress, antibiotics, alcohol	Weakness, indigestion, anxiety and irritability Sores on skin, rough skin Diarrhoea, swollen tongue, poor memory and concentration	Meat, fish, eggs, nuts, seeds, green leafy vegetables, mushrooms, tofu	Energy production from the digestion of fats, proteins and carbohydrates Improves circulation Reduces cholesterol Blood sugar regulation
B5 Pantothenic acid	Alone or with meals	B complex, folic acid, biotin	Stress, antibiotics	Impaired fat synthesis and energy production Vomiting and abdominal cramps, cramping, burning sensation in feet	Meat, poultry, fish, eggs, avocados, tomatoes, lentils, pulses and beans, sunflower seeds, mushrooms, whole grains	Nerve transmission, fat metabolism, immune system, stress response, formation of red blood cells Converting food into glucose Synthesizing cholesterol

Vitamin/ mineral	Best absorption	What helps	What hinders	Deficiency	Food source	Function
B6 Pyridoxine	Alone or with meals	B complex, magnesium, zinc	Stress, antibiotics, alcohol	Skin problems, i.e. acne Nervous system problems – depression, irritability, insomnia, poor coordination Impaired immunity Painful periods	Meat, fish, eggs, whole grains, dark leafy greens, bananas, carrots, potatoes, sunflower seeds, walnuts, avocados, pulses and beans, lentils	Protein digestion Nervous system function Blood cell and neurotransmitter formation
B12 Methyl- cobalamin	Alone or with meals	B complex, calcium	Stress, antibiotics, parasites, alcohol	More common in strict vegans/vegetarians and elderly Weight loss, fatigue, excessive bleeding, swollen and sore mouth and tongue, weakness, poor memory	Meat, liver, seafood, eggs	DNA synthesis Creation of red blood cells Development of brain and nerve cells
C Ascorbic acid	Alone or with meals	Hydrochloric acid in stomach	Heavy meals	Easy bruising, frequent infections, poor wound healing Loss of appetite Bleeding gums, muscle and joint pain	In all raw fresh fruit and vegetables	Helps the body form blood vessels, muscle and cartilage Helps prevent iron deficiency Immunity Antioxidant

FAT SOLUBLE VITAMINS

Vitamin/ mineral	Best absorption	What helps	What hinders	Deficiency	Food source	Function
A	Take with foods that have fat or oils	Zinc, C and E	Lack of bile	Dry eyes and skin, night blindness, throat and chest infections, poor wound healing, acne	Tomatoes, red bell peppers, beef, liver, milk, eggs, green leafy vegetables	Vision, cell division, reproduction, immunity
D	Take with foods that have fat or oils	Calcium, phosphorus, C and E	Lack of bile	Frequent illness and infections, tiredness, bone pain, back pain, depression, hair loss, poor wound healing, muscle pain	Salmon, sardines, herring, tinned tuna, egg yolk	Immunity, regulates mood and reduces depression
E	Take with foods that have fat or oils	Selenium, C	Lack of bile, ferric forms of iron, oxidized fats	Visual disturbance, muscle pain/weakness, difficulty walking	Almonds, spinach, avocados, kiwi fruit, broccoli, prawns	Helps the body use vitamin K, immunity antioxidant
K	Take with foods that have fat or oils	D, calcium	Lack of bile, too much vitamin E	Easy bruising, stools dark black and contain some blood	Green leafy vegetables – kale, collard greens, broccoli, spinach	Makes proteins for clotting and to build bones

MINERALS

Vitamin/mineral	Best absorption	What helps	What hinders	Deficiency	Food source	Function
Calcium	With protein	Magnesium, D hydrochloric acid in stomach	Tea, coffee, smoking	Weak, brittle nails, numbness and tingling in hand and face, muscle spasms, confusion or memory loss	Milk, cheese, yoghurt, kale, dark green leafy vegetables	Bone and teeth formation, nerve communication, muscle contraction
Magnesium	With protein at night	Calcium, B6, D, hydrochloric acid in stomach	Alcohol, tea, coffee, smoking	Muscle spasms, poor coordination, personality changes, loss of appetite, pins and needles, nausea	Avocados, dark chocolate, nuts, seeds, legumes, salmon, mackere, leafy greens	Blood pressure regulation, protein synthesis, blood glucose control, nerve function
Iron	With iron	C, hydrochloric acid in stomach	Oxalic acid, tannins in tea, coffee, smoking	Weak, tired, shortness of breath, anaemia	Shellfish, spinach liver, legumes, red meat, pumpkin seeds, quinoa	Helps convert blood sugar to energy, oxygenate the blood, immunity, blood production
Zinc	On an empty stomach – pm	B6, C, hydrochloric acid in stomach	Phytic acid, lead, copper, calcium, iron, tea, coffee	Unexplained weight loss, poor wound healing, diarrhoea, decreased sense of smell and taste	Oysters, shellfish, beef, pork, legumes, nuts, seeds	DNA synthesis, immunity, cell growth and division, protein production

What I find noticeable about this list is that the same factors that hinder absorption come up time after time: alcohol, smoking, antibiotics and stress. You will notice that the food sources for these vitamins and minerals are all whole, natural foods. You can't get your vitamins and minerals from processed food unless it has been fortified artificially. So, by limiting these and choosing whole foods as much as possible, it will mean you'll not only be healthier overall, but you'll reduce the likelihood of becoming deficient in vitamins and minerals.

You can target supplements to support specific functions or at particular times, for example, during times of stress. The time when you actually take the supplement is important due to their specific functions. As magnesium is a sleep aid, it is best to take this mineral at night.

Here are some common supplements you could try. Remember to try only one of these at a time so that you'll know if it works for you or not and to avoid any gastrointestinal upset.

When you need to de-stress

Ashwagandha

Ashwagandha is an ayurvedic herb found in parts of Northern Africa and India. It is classed as a nootropic as it can boost cognitive function, create a sense of calm and ease anxiety. It works by mimicking neurotransmitters in the brain that are responsible for feelings of wellbeing and boosting serotonin levels. Ashwagandha can support the body's inflammatory response, optimize blood pressure and improve memory. It can also help keep cortisol levels in check and reduce inflammation and increase muscle mass and strength in some individuals, particularly in those already on resistance training programs (Candelario et al., 2015). The best way to take it is as a supplement powder/tablets, as a tea or as an ashwagandha tincture. Research suggests that it works by regulating the chemical signalling within your nervous system, cutting off the pathway that recognizes stress and reducing your body's perception of fatigue. This is helpful because you can be physically tired (say, from a tough workout) but the adaptogen reduces how you experience fatigue, making you feel less tired. Ashwagandha can interact with some medications and conditions, so (as with all supplements) consult your doctor before taking it.

Holy basil

Holy basil (*Ocimum sanctum* or tulsi) is native to Southeast Asia and is said to reduce stress and anxiety, thanks to the antidepressant and anti-anxiety-like compounds it contains. It mimics the actions of diazepam and other antidepressant drugs. The best way to take it is as a tea or a supplement powder/tablet.

Other studies have shown that, when taken in conjunction with milk thistle, holy basil can support liver protection. If you consume a lot of alcohol, you will need to support your liver. Whilst cutting down or eliminating alcohol altogether is the best option, the combination of holy basil and milk thistle could work well.

Lactobacillus rhamnosus

This is a probiotic naturally found in the gut but sometimes lacking in those with poor gut health. It produces the enzyme lactase, which breaks down lactose – found in dairy products – into lactic acid. You can also find it in yoghurt, kefir and any other fermented products. It's a beneficial strain of probiotic for IBS and if you take it as a probiotic that includes the strain rhamnosus, it is said to modulate stress and anxiety.

When you need to sleep

Valerian root

Valerian root (*Valeriana officinalis*) is an ayurvedic herb native to Asia and Europe. Valerian contains valerenic acid, isovaleric acid and a number of antioxidants. These are the active constituents that reduce anxiety by inhibiting gamma-aminobutyric acid (GABA) breakdown in the brain, resulting in feelings of calm. Anti-anxiety medications like Valium and Xanax work in the same way.

The antioxidants hesperidin and linarin found in the root of valerian have sedative and hypnotic properties, which is why valerian tea can be an excellent sleep aid.

Lemon balm

Lemon balm is a herb from the mint family that has been used since the Middle Ages to reduce stress and anxiety, aid sleep and ease indigestion, gas and bloating. You can use lemon balm tea as a supplement, but make sure you use 2 tea bags for a therapeutic dose.

L-Theanine

L-Theanine is an amino acid found in green and black tea and some mushrooms, but you can take it as a supplement. It increases alpha waves, which make you relax and help with anxiety and sleep.

Magnesium glycinate

This type of magnesium enhances sleep patterns and is beneficial for cardiovascular health as it helps to lower blood pressure.

Phosphatidylserine

This stabilizes the circadian rhythm, our body's way of knowing when to be awake and when to sleep. Studies have shown that phosphatidylserine reduces as we age, so supplementation can be useful.

TOP TIP 🖊

Add 2 large cups of magnesium flakes to a warm bath or a foot bath/bowl if you don't have a bath.

At times of low energy

Rhodiola rosea

An adaptogen and nootropic, this helps the body adapt to stress by reducing fatigue and exhaustion. Rhodiola rosea has over 140 active ingredients to balance mood by regulating cortisol levels. Excess cortisol can impair memory function, affect blood pressure, blood sugar and metabolism. Rhodiola rosea can help those suffering with adrenal fatigue by increasing energy and concentration.

Acetyl-L-Carnitine

This plays an important role in energy production by transporting fatty acids into your mitochondria so they can be oxidized (Flanagan et al., 2010).

D-ribose

D-ribose naturally occurs in the cells, and particularly in the mitochondria. D-ribose supplements have been shown to improve cellular processes when there is mitochondrial dysfunction and improve energy production.

B vitamins

These convert the food we consume into ATP. There are eight B vitamins and each has a slightly different function. To cover them all, take a B vitamin complex supplement.

Selenium and iron

Selenium is essential for thyroid activity. Iron is vital in the cellular process to convert food into ATP.

Vitamins C and E

Both vitamin C and vitamin E are powerful antioxidants that help neutralize free radicals.

Alpha Lipoic Acid

Is involved in energy metabolism and fights off the effects of free radicals. It can help slow down cellular damage.

Coenzyme Q10 (CoQ10)

An antioxidant that decreases with age. Its core function is to generate energy within the cells and help produce ATP. Although it is found in meat, nuts and fish it is not enough to increase levels within the body, so supplementation is necessary.

Resveratrol

A polyphenol (micronutrient in plants) that can help promote ATP production. It is shown to promote mitochondrial production and recycles dysfunctional mitochondria. It is found in red wine.

When you keep getting ill

Astragalus

Astragalus is used to promote longevity, fight inflammation, strengthen the immune system and treat heart and kidney conditions.

Astragalus differs from other adaptogens as it's the only natural substance to contain cycloastragenol. Cycloastragenol has anti-stress, anti-ageing and anti-bacterial properties.

Reishi mushrooms

Like astragalus, reishi mushrooms are a popular choice for supporting the immune system. A type of fungus that grows in hot and humid regions of Asia, these mushrooms have been used in Eastern medicine for thousands of years. Reishi mushrooms can be eaten fresh, but it's common to see them ground down into a powder form for easier and more convenient consumption. Whichever way you take reishi, it's important to note that they should only be eaten for medication and not consistently as part of a diet.

Reishi are full of antioxidants, which combat oxidative damage caused by free radicals. Some strains of reishi have even been found to alter inflammation pathways in white blood cells, which help to fight infection and cancer.

TOP TIP 🖊

Make sure if you are taking any medication that you check first with your doctor or healthcare professional. Certain drugs such as warfarin can react with many of the listed nutrients. If your doctor doesn't know, you can speak to many of the reputable supplement or healthcare companies who are trained to discuss drug/nutrient interactions.

David was an ultra-athlete who loved nothing better than pushing himself to his physical limit, but he came to see me complaining of loose stools, bloating, poor sleep and aches and pains in his joints. He wanted to take part in some intensive races, but it was evident that his tenacity and dedication were taking a toll on his body.

One of the reasons David couldn't sleep was the feeling of restlessness in his body, particularly his legs. He had a twitchy eye, especially when he was tired, and he struggled to recover after his exercise.

When we looked at David's diet, it was clear that he wasn't eating the right nutritious foods for his needs. A lot of his food was made up of snacks and meals on the go. He didn't take any time to chew his food, so it was likely his body wasn't absorbing the nutrients well enough, leaving him depleted.

Before we looked at supplementing David's diet, we made some changes. We added more fibre-rich foods, such as oats, rye bread and brown rice to bulk the stools and increased his protein, as when we calculated how much David was getting per day it wasn't sufficient for the amount of exercise he was doing. Finally, we made sure all David's meals were being eaten sitting down while he was relaxed to improve digestion and absorption. Only then did we start to look at supplementation. Because of the twitchiness and poor sleep, we started by prescribing a magnesium glycinate supplement. This contained vitamin C to reduce tiredness and fatigue and B vitamins to support his energy production.

When David came to see me for his follow-up appointment, he said he felt like a different person. His energy had increased and he was able to increase his running times. He'd even landed a personal best. His sleep had improved, and the twitching and restlessness had stopped.

What about superfoods?

Superfoods contain high levels of certain micronutrients and can be used to supplement your diet. Superfoods have gained a lot of press in recent years, both good and bad, and it's all become a bit confusing. Is there such a thing as a superfood? And if so, what makes a food super?

Whatever you want to call them, it's true that some foods are more nutritious than others. A food could be classified as a 'superfood' (Wolfe, 2009) if:

- It has six or more unique characteristics.
- It contains bioactive compounds that support the healthy functioning of the body.
- It contains important antioxidants, such as vitamins A, C and E, flavonoids, selenium, ß-carotene, zinc, lycopene, albumin, uric acid, bilirubin, coenzyme Q10 and polyphenols like anthocyanidin.

As well as taking micronutrients in the form of supplements, you might be able to supplement your diet using some of the foods below:

Mushrooms

Mushrooms are full of BIG nutrition because they not only support the brain, the immune system *and* the gut, but they have a major superpower: they are one of the few foods that can convert ultraviolet light from the sun into vitamin D. They contain high amounts of the antioxidants ergothioneine and glutathione. If you can get hold of them, the following mushrooms are particularly good for energy:

Cordyceps

This is one of the best mushrooms for energy as it mimics molecularly ATP, our energy currency, and actually helps facilitate its production. Interestingly, in 1993 three Chinese women in the Beijing Olympics were accused of doping after improving their personal bests, however they were tested for banned substances but their results came back negative. When they were asked about how they managed to achieve such a feat, they said apart from their altitude training they had created a special elixir that contained the Cordyceps mushroom, which they believe led to their success. We can't underestimate the power of just mushrooms alone in energy production and endurance (Yesalis, 2002).

Shiitake

Shiitake mushrooms, which we tend to associate with Asian cuisine, are great for energy due to their high broad-spectrum vitamin B content. B vitamins are vital cofactors to make our energy. As a reminder, stress depletes our B vitamins, so mushrooms can provide a good support if you are undergoing a stressful, low-energy period. They can be taken in capsules and powders, but they are best consumed in their fresh form.

Lion's mane

Called Lion's mane as they do resemble the incredible shagginess of the mane of a lion, this mushroom contains nootropic properties, which studies show may improve overall mood. They have cognitive properties, such as boosting focus and memory. Lion's mane mushrooms contain BDNF – brain-derived neurotrophic factor – a protein that is neuroprotective, i.e. supports brain health.

Chaga

This mushroom is very high in SOD – the enzyme super-oxide dismutase, which kills the naughty free radical superoxide and prevents DNA damage to the body. They are rich in beta glucans, which is great for activating the immune system. Chaga is an adaptogen, which can help your body change its physiological state, so if you are feeling really stressed, chaga could help the body reverse that state.

Berries

Pomegranate, berries, blueberries, raspberries, strawberries, goji berry, grapes and acai berries all contain antioxidants and anthocyanins, which give these fruits their electric rainbow-like colours. Blueberries, raspberries and blackberries are said to have the highest antioxidant activity, followed by pomegranates (Kelly et al., 2008). Berries are incredibly versatile and are great in smoothies, over porridge, as snacks with a piece of protein, made into compote, drizzled into full-fat Greek yoghurt or even spread onto toast with nut butter. If you feel daring, try and make sweet potato toasts topped with nut butter and mashed raspberries.

Nuts and seeds

Walnuts, almonds and other tree nuts contain everything you need for a healthy balanced diet. Healthy fats, Omega 3s, plant protein, fibre, the list is endless. Yet many of us either don't think about including nuts and seeds in our diets or avoid due to the incorrect press about how 'fatty' nuts can be. If you can include one thing in your diet, unless you have a nut allergy, make it these. They are super snacks, keeping you full for a much longer period of time. If you are concerned about giving nuts to your family, you can opt for ground flaxseed, linseeds, chia seeds, or grind nuts down with a pestle and mortar to sprinkle onto breakfasts, vegetables and salads.

Pulses

Pulses are the most underrated, inexpensive and under-utilized superfood. All types of beans, lentils and peas are superfoods, except for shop-bought baked beans, and they pack a real punch in terms of nutrients. They contain protein, fibre, fats and a ton of vitamins and minerals. Some studies suggest that it's the reason why the Japanese, Swedish and Mediterranean people live longer (Darmadi-Blackberry et al., 2004). Just remember hummus, dhal, black bean chilli, bean quesadillas and homemade baked beans are all great options for including pulses in your diet. Tinned and pre-prepared pulses are quicker options if you don't want to spend time cooking them.

Seaweed

Seaweed contains lots of antioxidants, vitamins A, C and E and iodine, crucial for the health of the thyroid. Spirulina and chlorella are both members of the algae family and contain protein and an abundance of vitamins and minerals. They are said to support blood sugar control (Hozayen et al., 2016). If seaweed isn't your thing, try sprinkling nori flakes over your salads or eating thin seaweed sheets you can buy in most supermarkets. If you get a takeaway sushi meal ask for the seaweed salad too, it's delicious.

KEY ACTIONS IN STEP 4: ENERGIZE WITH SUPPLEMENTS

- When supplementing with nutrients, check with your doctor or nutritionist if you take prescription drugs.
- Only take supplements once you have started to make changes to your diet, gut health, sleep and exercise.
- Check when you should take supplements to maximize absorption. Certain supplements should be taken with others or at a certain time of day.

- Watch out for fillers and binders in supplements and always buy from a reputable source.
- Don't forget that superfoods contain high levels of certain micronutrients and can often be used to supplement your diet.

Step 5

Harness the Power of Your Brain
Managing the Mind

> Almost everything will work again if you
> unplug for a few minutes, including you.

Anne Lamott

If you were around in the 1980s then you'll remember that CFS (then known as ME) had the nickname 'yuppie flu'. The implication was clear: lazy young professionals were growing tired of working hard and as a result developed a psychological 'illness' that mysteriously made them feel constantly tired. Most of the press at the time insinuated that it was very much all in the mind, and anyone with ME was seen to be weak and unable to cope with life. Since then, despite much research into CFS that shows specific changes in immunity with clear diagnostic markers, there is still a perception that long-term fatigue is partly 'in the mind'. So, is this true?

It might surprise you to know that my answer is no . . . and yes.

No, because fatigue absolutely does exist and you are not imagining it. Research shows that CFS sufferers show reduced mitochondrial function and other biological markers that prove they are not making their illness up. In fact, Dr Ron Davis at Stanford University said in his 2019 study on CFS, 'There is scientific evidence that this disease is not a fabrication of a patient's mind. We clearly see a difference in the way healthy and chronic fatigue syndrome immune cells process stress.'

So, if you have ever been dismissed by a medical practitioner or told your tiredness is a figment of your imagination, please know that it is not.

That said, there is a strong correlation between long-term fatigue and the functioning of your brain. Your mind – in other words, your thought patterns, cognitive function, personality and character traits – could have a profound effect on how tired you are. For this reason, managing your mind can be the final piece of the jigsaw puzzle in fixing fatigue.

The power of the brain

In 1984, Russian Anatoly Karpov was set to play fellow Russian and newbie on the scene Garry Kasparov at the World Chess Championships in Moscow. The rivals turned out to be incredibly well matched, and after five months, the score had reached five wins for Karpov, three wins for Kasparov and a grand total of forty draws. By this time, the adjudicator had serious concerns about the players' health. Karpov had turned up looking worryingly emaciated and it later turned out he had lost 10 kilograms (22 pounds) during the match, without seemingly doing anything at all. Eventually, the adjudicator called off the contest.

How had Karpov lost so much weight? After all, he was only sitting down all day. The fact is that, just like sport where weight loss can be a by-product of intense training, a mental game such as chess can be physically exhausting. In fact, chess players can burn up to 6,000 calories in a professional game.

If something as cerebral as chess, which requires careful, well-thought-out decisions, can be a drain on energy, it follows that anything that uses our brain can be just as tiring. This could include being overstimulated, overthinking, worrying, regularly having poor self-esteem, feeling anxious, thinking negatively or making too many decisions.

In this step we're going to look at the mental activities that could be making you tired and suggest some changes that will preserve your energy and manage how you feel about your symptoms.

TOP TIP 🖉

Don't forget it's not just our bodies that need rest but our brains too. Take some form of brain rest every single day.

Avoid overstimulation

Feeling overstimulated is becoming increasingly common. When our senses are heightened and stimulated, we can experience what is known as 'sensory overload' – and it can leave us feeling irritable and overwhelmed. When our brain has to compete with lots of different sensory information gleaned from the external environment, it cannot process it all at once or know which information to prioritize.

Below are some of the things that can contribute to sensory overload and some solutions to reduce their impact:

Technology
Set tech times in your day and avoid using tech outside of these.

Light
Have morning natural light, ideally outside, and use red/amber light in the evenings to elicit sleep rather than blue light, which is better for productivity.

Noise
Don't always have sound in your ears. Go for walks without a podcast or listening to music, switch off the TV, be comfortable with silence.

Social media
The big brain drain. Figure out your purpose for using it and identify appropriate-length social media time slots.

Large gatherings

Avoid if they drain your energy or attend for a sweet spot number of hours.

Make sure you take regular breaks from sensory experiences, especially if you are already tired. FSD – Fatigue, Sleep deprivation and Dehydration – can exacerbate the issue, so ensure you follow Step 3 (see page 162) earlier in the book to build a good sleep routine. Also ensure you drink plenty of water throughout the day and remind yourself to take brain breaks. You could use these to unwind by:

- moving
- writing
- reading
- meditating or breathing
- or doing absolutely nothing!

One of my clients who struggled with sensory overload was Hilary. She came to my clinic complaining of exhaustion, depression and Hashimoto's disease, an autoimmune condition that can cause underactive thyroid. She worked in a stressful corporate job and was fed up with feeling flat, dejected and unmotivated. She just couldn't seem to find joy in anything she was doing.

On the surface it looked like Hilary was eating a healthy diet, with lots of pre-packaged raw salads, soups, fish and steamed vegetables. However, I noticed that she wasn't consuming any carbohydrates or healthy fats and wasn't eating enough protein. It was when I asked about Hilary's lifestyle and routine, though, that we got to the bottom of her low energy. As soon as she got up in the morning Hilary would check her phone, and she would continue to check social media and answer emails throughout the day. She rarely took a break as she felt like she had to be constantly on the move. She was draining her own brain energy without realizing it.

We started by adding some nutritious foods to Hilary's diet. These included complex carbohydrates, such as sweet potatoes, brown rice and oats. We increased healthy fats to support brain function, such as flaxseed, chia seeds and tree nuts like almonds. I asked her to switch all her raw vegetables to homemade cooked vegetables to support her digestion, as her gut was having to work far harder at breaking down the raw vegetables. She very quickly started to feel better. However, the biggest change to Hilary's energy came by calming down her brain and giving it time to rest. She switched her frantic, long walks for stretching, slow-flow yoga and meditation.

Manage mind chatter

Even though the brain is classed as an organ and not a muscle, it can get chemically tired just thinking too much. Your thoughts really do dictate how you feel and your internal chatter has the ability to fuel or starve your brain of energy. If you have a busy mind – perhaps you're an overthinker, a dreamer, creative or entrepreneur – finding a way to process or offload those thoughts to ensure your mental energy and performance is maintained will be important. There is a lot of emphasis placed on eradicating negative thoughts these days, but with internal chatter thoughts can be at both ends of the spectrum, good and bad – or somewhere in between.

We have on average around 6,200 thoughts a day, and it might surprise you to know that as many as 80 per cent of these are negative. Even more surprisingly, up to 95 per cent are repeats of the day before (Tseng and Poppenk, 2020). So, if you had a stressful day, it's likely that you'll repeat many of those stressful thoughts tomorrow. What a waste of energy!

Whilst it's relatively easy to reduce external stimuli that can affect our brains, such as technology, lights and noise, our internal chatter is far harder to fix. We drain our own brain energy very easily. I realized recently in my clinic that, just like Hilary, many of my clients presenting with fatigue and exhaustion were draining their own brain energy without realizing it, not only through poor diet and a sedentary lifestyle, but through how they were thinking.

One way of controlling mind chatter is to write. In her brilliant book *The Artist's Way*, Julia Cameron suggests writing three pages of notes every day as soon as you get up. She calls these 'morning pages'. Just write three pages, no more or no less, about anything that springs to mind – it can be big, small or trivial. What's important is the process of clearing your mind so you can start the day afresh without worry, stress or any other emotion you may be experiencing hijacking your day.

Morning pages allow you to notice any themes coming up. Which thoughts are recurring and what are they trying to tell you? You may find within this a new career is trying to present itself, a hobby, an idea or an issue that may need resolving. The problem with thoughts is that often you don't make any progress with them. It's like going round a roundabout and never being able to take the right road. This means your energy is being drained for no reason at all as you are unable to reach a conclusion or solution. Morning pages might just remove those thoughts for you.

Conserve brain energy

So, what can we do to conserve our brain energy and avoid mental fatigue?

There are some small changes you can make to stop your brain becoming a serious energy leak.

Keep glucose levels steady

When glucose levels drop because the brain has used up all its fuel, lowered glucose levels raise ATP, which blocks dopamine. As we know, dopamine is our reward chemical, which makes us feel good. A lack of dopamine means we are less likely to stay motivated and focused on the task we are working on, simply because we don't feel good doing it (Martin, 2018). For this reason, ensuring glucose levels stay balanced is important to avoid mental fatigue. Say you have an important interview. If you have a rushed breakfast of sugary cereal, miss your train and arrive late to the interview, you will already have depleted a lot of your glucose. If on the other hand you have a protein-filled breakfast, leave plenty of time for your train and arrive in a calm state, you will be mentally better prepared to perform at your best. Sugar is damaging to the brain and research shows that it shrinks and damages nerve connections, making it far harder to learn, develop and remember new things (Edwards, 2016).

TOP TIP 🖊

Sugar comes in many forms, not just the white table sugar you can buy. Sweeteners, agave syrup and honey all have the same effect on your glucose levels. However, lower GI (glycaemic options) like stevia, dates and apple sauce can still provide a sweet hit.

Building a second brain

Sometimes the sheer volume of things swirling around in our minds can drain our brains. It is that feeling of fullness that may cause a slight brain ache or head tension, which is down to having way too much to think about. Sometimes, this can cause us to feel agitated, stressed and irritable because the build-up of tasks in our heads feels too overwhelming.

There is a solution. Build a second brain. The difference? It's a digital one. If your current brain feels full to the brim, create a new second brain where you can download all your information into. Sounds simple? Well, according to Tiago Forte, author of *Building a Second Brain*, who created the concept, it really is. He believes if you want to become more productive and reach your full creative potential, this is the best way to do it.

We consume so much information on a daily basis and this is a digital online note-taking system that captures anything that resonates with you that you read, watch and listen to. Trello, Notion, your notes section in your phone, a simple Excel spreadsheet or Word document all work well. This filtering system allows you to better organize your thoughts. This new headspace can house all your information in one safe area so you don't forget anything, reducing overload and stress. Not only will this free up space in your current brain, but your thoughts will become more organized and systematic.

You may be wondering why this is important. We know our brains use up the most energy in our body. If we can actively take steps to reduce this, we won't feel so cognitively tired. Having one brain is fine but two is even better if you want to supercharge your productivity and potential. Take start-ups. Start-ups have a far greater chance of succeeding with a co-founder. See your second brain as your co-founder, necessary for optimal productivity and performance.

How you go about it ultimately determines your success. The planning and organizing part is key. Once you read this book, your mind may be spinning by the sheer amount of information. I hope that it is broken down into easy-to-understand bite-size chunks, but even these small snippets of information will naturally get your brain thinking and excited to start. By building an external outside brain, you can extract the most important parts of this book and then summarize them so that you know exactly what you need to learn from it and action. This is known as progressive summarization. It's a summary of a summary of a summary distilled down into tiny manageable chunks:

- Note down in your second brain what it is that has resonated with you most – no more than five things, e.g. adding nutrients into food is better than cutting out food groups.
- With these five things, can you distil these down further? e.g. nutrient toppers can be added to food to increase nutrient density.
- Are you now left with a goal that you can easily action? e.g. add a nutrient topper such as a large spoonful of nuts and seeds to breakfast every morning.

You can then create this small list of actions as a starting point and put it up somewhere visible, such as on a Post-it on the fridge.

GUIDANCE

- Identify what is consuming your own brain's thoughts, such as too many ideas. Is there a pattern? What keeps swirling around your brain?
- Figure out the best way to download that information. Is it in the notes section of your phone? A spreadsheet? An online digital board? Apps like Trello, Evernote, Microsoft OneNote, Bear and Notion are all useful tools too.
- Start storing and assess the impact that having a co-founder is having on your mental energy.

Once you start to get into the habit of downloading your thoughts and information into one safe space, how do you feel? Do you have less overwhelm and brain fog?

TOP TIP ✏️

Once you have tried this out, revisit this
section in a month's time. Note how your
brain feels:

....
....
....
....
....
....
....
....

You may be wondering how I have built my second brain? The
answer to this is very simple, and it is certainly a work-in-
progress. I use the notes section in my phone to categorize
everything I think. My brain has a tendency to go into overdrive, especially when I am creatively stretched and excited. By
noting things down as I think about them, my brain doesn't
have to worry about forgetting that action or thought. My second brain however does need to evolve as my workload and
family responsibilities increase. I know it can be even better to
maximize my learning and productivity but just by making a
small start I am already reaping the cognitive benefits.

Avoid multitasking

Multitasking is one hell of a brain drain. According to neuro-scientists, trying to juggle too many tasks at once causes problems with memory and concentration. If the two tasks are very simple and make sense to do at the same time, such as reading the paper whilst sipping a cup of tea, that's fine. But when you combine challenging tasks like a difficult work project and sending an important email, the brain is less able to cope. It's only when we practise deep work-focus without distraction or enter a state of flow where we dedicate a chunk of time just to one activity, that we see results because the mind isn't trying to do lots of things at once. When this happens, we not only get a happier brain, but we're far more productive.

Breathe correctly

It is vital to breathe oxygen into our system and take carbon dioxide away. There are two types of breathing – nasal and mouth. Nasal is more efficient as mouth breathing is less so and makes us more prone to infection. However, mouth exhalation can be beneficial because you get 20 per cent more oxygen when breathing through the nose and not through the mouth. When you breathe properly, you can alter the chemistry of your body and produce intentional physiological responses (Wim Hof).

THREE SIMPLE BREATHING EXERCISES TO TRY

- Double the exhale – breathe in for 4 and out for 8.
- 444 breathing – breathe in for 4, hold for 4 and then slowly exhale out for 4 via the mouth.
- Equal breathing – breathe in for the same amount of time as you exhale, e.g. in for 8 and out for 8.

TOP TIP 🖉

After exercise, take 5–10 minutes just to lie down and breathe to help with recovery.

Manage your thoughts

Controlling how and what we think might sound impossible, but it's actually easier than you think. With a little practice, you can learn to notice unhelpful thoughts and stop them from draining your energy. This is particularly helpful if you are struggling with long-term fatigue. To do this, use the ACE acronym:

A = Acknowledge thoughts and feelings (as far as possible without self-judgement). Try naming the thought process (e.g. 'There's an anxious/worried/frustrated thought,') and notice where you feel the emotion in your body.

C = Connect with your body. Ground your feet into the floor, stretch your back, press your hands and fingers together. Bring your focus of attention to your physical being as encapsulating your thoughts and feelings.

E = Engage with the world around you. Notice four things you can see, four things you can hear and four things you can touch.

Know your personality

In Chapter 1 (see page 40) we learnt that some people process emotions more acutely than others, and that these people can be classed as HSPs, or Highly Sensitive People. For these people, tiredness can be a very real result of overthinking, ruminating and ongoing worry. Whether you're an introvert or an extrovert can determine how much energy your brain uses and when. This is why understanding your personality and where your energy goes is crucial for fixing psychological or emotional fatigue.

If you're a Highly Sensitive Person, you'll be particularly attuned to the feelings of people around you. You might feel misunderstood, not only in the workplace, but in general society. Managing your brain energy will mean prioritizing the mental activities that are important to you. That means your social interactions will be about the quality of the connection, not the quantity, and meeting people with whom you truly connect. When you connect with the right people, this in itself creates positive feelings of wellbeing and increases our energy. Notice this next time you surround yourself with friends. How do you feel after certain interactions? Positively or negatively charged?

It's important to have boundaries. Without strict boundaries, your energy can be depleted very quickly. Knowing the types of people that understand you and allow your boundaries to remain intact is key. This, coupled with giving yourself full permission to recharge as much as you need, is incredibly important. Being unapologetically you and not changing around others according to their needs will sustain your precious energy.

Coping strategies for HSPs

- Choose jobs where you will thrive in the working environment and preferably where you can work flexibly. The culture must align with your values.
- Find fellow HSPs to hang out with so you feel understood. Trust me, there are lots out there!
- Take proper time out to recharge. Think about how many hours or days a week you need to spend alone and strike the right balance between being sociable with topping up your energy levels alone.
- Find time to be creative and prioritize doing things you love. Studies show that we are normally more creative in the afternoons than in the mornings, when our brains are slightly more frazzled, as we have less focus and are more likely to allow our minds to drift (Weith and Zacks, 2011).
- Say no to anything that might compromise your energy.

Look after your gut

As we know, the brain and gut are inextricably linked. But there's even some evidence to suggest that your gut determines your personality. If you find social situations draining, there's a chance you can change your personality type through your gut microbiota. According to recent research, improving the diversity of your microbes in your gut will help turn you into a more socially confident person.

Katerina Johnson, PhD from the Department of Experimental Psychology at Oxford University used the International Personality Item Pool, consisting of 50 items to assess personality traits based on the 'five-factor model of personality'.

The results showed people with more extensive social networks were more likely to have greater bacterial diversity. Therefore, socially active individuals may have healthier guts! This links to past research conducted into the same strains of bacteria found in autism. Those with lower microbial diversity were associated with higher levels of stress and anxiety. This indicates that if we look after our guts, it will have an impact on our overall personality, energy and wellbeing. I know when I eat well and follow a healthy lifestyle, I feel calmer, I have energy, I am more sociable, and I feel generally happier and more content.

As we have seen, our minds can deplete our energy in many different ways. Protecting your brain energy is key to good health. This comes down to what you fuel it with, how you process external stimulation and your thoughts. But as we now know, even though science is in its very early stages, your gut/brain connection may be able to dictate some of your personality traits. So, by feeding your gut the right nourishing foods, this can really ensure both your gut and brain are working optimally.

KEY ACTIONS IN STEP 5: HARNESS THE POWER OF YOUR BRAIN

- Avoid overstimulation by taking regular breaks from tech, noise and social media.
- Manage your mind chatter by writing 'morning pages' every day.
- Know what type of personality you are and establish boundaries to protect your brain energy.
- Look after your gut by revisiting Step 2 (see page 144) – the microbiome in your gut can affect your personality.
- Incorporate regular breath work into your daily routine to conserve your brain energy.
- Use thought management techniques like the ACE acronym to avoid spiralling into anxiety or depressive thoughts.

Epilogue

Measuring Success

Success is the product of daily habits –
not once-in-a-lifetime transformations.

James Clear

As with anything, sustaining a habit for the long term can be hard. We can get distracted, lose sight of the original goal or swap the habit for something newer and shinier before it has become ingrained in our psyches. The hardest thing about implementing the practices you've learnt in this book isn't starting off – it's keeping going. Fixing fatigue with ongoing lifestyle changes is particularly hard because when you are exhausted, finding motivation is even more difficult.

The first thing to know is that if you want to improve your energy, it has to become your number one focus. Maybe not forever, but for the time being at least. It takes on average 66 days to instil a new habit, but it may take less or more time than this. The trick is not to give up. Making a habit easy and simple to ingrain into your daily routine will increase your chances of success. After that, you should not only find that they've become part of your life, but you should have started to see some positive changes.

Measuring success

Tangible goals, like losing weight, are easy to measure – you can see your results reflected in the scales or as your clothes get looser. But how do you measure energy levels? There simply isn't an easy way to measure how tired you are. In this case, rather than setting definitive goals, it's best to set therapeutic aims. These aims are nurturing and clear in their purpose rather than restrictive and punishing. Here are some examples:

- Have enough energy to complete a 2k run or walk.
- Improve my gut microbiome so that my pain and bloating stops.
- Develop better sleep hygiene so I have more energy throughout the day.
- Reduce sugar to stabilize blood sugar levels to avoid energy dips.
- Eat a portion of cruciferous vegetables every day to improve my magnesium levels.

By setting one of these aims and working on it every single day without pressure and without overthinking it, you can make your goals a part of you rather than feeling forced and restricted.

A different way of measuring your success is to use the scale of fatigue on page 25. Your tiredness might still vary from day to day, so measure yourself over the course of a week to see if there is any improvement.

Another question is how can you stay accountable when the changes feel too hard to stick to? Finding willpower in those cold winter months or during a stressful period can be particularly hard. Kelly McGonigal PhD, author of *The Willpower Instinct*, describes the ability to do what you need to do, even if part of you doesn't want to. The key here is when you don't want to do it. There are of course days when you would much rather get a takeaway than cook from scratch or scroll on your phone a bit longer rather than get to bed an hour earlier, but your mind and body will thank you for it if you stick to your plan.

It is all down to long-lasting behavioural change. Habits are interesting. Some habits are autonomic, such as getting into the car and buckling up your seatbelt. This could be because we associate the seatbelt with safety and so it feels important, but it's most likely that we have done it so often that as soon as we get into the car we are triggered – it feels natural to do it and we don't even have to think about it. Making our lifestyle habits as easy and natural as this is the goal – we want them to feel automatic.

The seven actions for good habits over the page will help you get started on your goals. Remember, there's no punishment for 'falling off the wagon' – each day is a new day and the rewards will happen even if you let things slip once or twice. You know *why* you need to make these changes, so this is about *how*:

Action 1: Start small

Action 2: Keep it simple

Action 3: Be prepared

Action 4: Know your triggers and note them down

Action 5: Be realistic

Action 6: Make it obvious

Action 7: Embrace boredom

ACTION 1: Start small

Choose your focus. What are your goals and what do you want to focus on? It might be to have more energy, improve your gut health or get better-quality sleep. The key is to not try and make too many changes all at once. When we switch from one goal to another, a neurochemical switch is ignited in the brain that uses up key brain nutrients and depletes our precious glucose stores. Pick one achievable thing to start off with and stick to it for a period of time.

ACTION 2: Keep it simple

If you're working long hours, looking after a family and feeling tired and stressed, you need to keep your new habits simple. You can always aim higher once you are firmly into your new lifestyle but make these first steps easy to achieve. This means making sure home-cooked meals only take 15 minutes and don't require endless and difficult-to-buy ingredients. Have a good store cupboard with cheap and quick things to prepare, such as pre-packaged quinoa, brown rice and lentil packs, a variety of beans and tinned vegetables such as sweetcorn.

ACTION 3: Be prepared

Dr Darria Long in her study showed that 70 per cent of individuals who put chocolate out of reach didn't eat it. Her ethos is not to focus on willpower but to design things differently. So, think about how you can take better control of your surroundings and environment to create healthier habits and a better chance of success.

Plan what you are going to do. Pick a day of the week to decide what you are going to eat for the week and make a list of what you need to get. Now decide how you are going to implement the changes. Do you need to:

- Create a new shopping list. Where will you shop? What day will you place the order? Can you save healthy favourites in your online account? What can you cut back on that you no longer need? How can you redistribute these funds for healthy items?
- Diarize reminders in your phone for shops, classes, workouts and meal prep. Where and how can you notice them? How can they not become a distractor?
- Book any classes through an app. Which app will you download and when?
- Download any useful apps. What do you need support with? Sleep? Nutrition? Breathing?
- Use tracking tools (although not calorie trackers) to track your micronutrient intake or other useful nutrients.

- Tell people what you are doing to stay accountable and ideally get them to join you. Who will be on your team? Who is positive and encouraging and will keep you going when you hit a wall?

ACTION 4: *Know your triggers and note them down*
Understand your weak spots, write them down and note a solution next to them. Some examples might be:

- If you are stressed, instead of overthinking have a bath, a massage or do yoga.
- If you are planning on eating with friends and you're tempted to eat junk food, enlist their help by getting them to cook a meal from scratch instead. Your sphere of influence and the people around you are hugely important in determining whether you can change your lifestyle or not.
- If you're hungry and irritable, instead of reaching for a sugar high make sure you always have a healthy snack and water on you to keep energy levels up, even in the car.
- If you find that during emotional times you eat, change your environment instead. Go for a walk, visit a friend or relative or do something fun that doesn't involve food.

ACTION 5: Be realistic

Are you a new mum? A busy career person? Juggling a lot of balls or recovering from an illness? Don't try to make too many changes at once or put too much pressure on yourself. You could try stacking habits. This is when we layer new habits on top of old ones, for example, doing some deep breathing or squats (new habit) while making a cup of tea (old habit). Over time, every time you do the old habit it will remind you to do the new one.

ACTION 6: Make it obvious

See page 126 for some fascinating insight into nudge theory, but making it obvious is basically about doing something that ensures you remember to take action. This could be making your healthy snack visible in the fridge so you remember to eat it or having a bottle of water by your bed to hydrate first thing in the morning.

ACTION 7: Embrace boredom

So many of our decisions in life are made in a hurry or when we are stressed, tired, hungry or emotional. But what if we just got better at embracing being bored? No scrolling, no TV, no sounds, just being. What if we were able to just let our minds wander without needing a distraction? To just be and rest more? By embracing boredom, we begin to make clearer, conscious, healthier choices. According to neuroscientists, boredom is achieved when we go into default mode, that state that's a little bit beyond consciousness into the subconscious. This is where we spark creativity. If we entered this land a little more often, daydreamed and relaxed more, perhaps our likelihood of success would be greater. We'd have less stress, more rest, more conscious decision making and a calmer approach to life. When the body relaxes and the cortisol levels go down, our internal homeostasis reaches a better equilibrium state. Constant sympathetic system dominance isn't healthy and certainly impacts our energy levels. This is where your body is in fight or flight mode. In low-stress individuals, we switch between the sympathetic and parasympathetic system via the HPA axis – the hypothalamic pituitary adrenal axis. In chronically stressed individuals, the HPA axis becomes desensitized, creating sympathetic system dominance.

GAME CHANGING TOP FIVE TAKEAWAYS FROM *THE ENERGY FIX*

- Good nutrition starts with adding things *into* your diet, not taking things away. Then in time you can make swaps that will increase the nutrients in your food. Find out what foods work for you and your body.
- Never normalize tiredness – being tired all the time isn't normal. Don't delay – seek help.

- Become your own private investigator to discover the root cause of your symptoms.
- Eat as much variety as possible for increased bacterial diversity. Avoid beige!
- Head to the NOCO Health platform if you need further help and support.

Energy is finite. Just like money in the bank, if you spend faster than you earn, you will quite simply run out. You don't want to do that because your energy is the most precious thing you own. The reason to eat well is because you need the right nutrients to create the right chemical reactions in your body to produce energy. Without energy, you cannot love life, look after your family, achieve at work or relate to your loved ones. It needs to be nurtured and protected in order to be maintained and sustained. Do not accept low or no energy as normal – it is a sign that your body is trying to tell you something. The best thing you can do for yourself is listen. Improving your energy and fixing your fatigue for good can be within your control – all the tools are in this book. And once you focus on your energy, everything else will fall into place.

Personal letter

You may be wondering how I am today and whether tiredness is still a problem for me? I am really pleased to say that I am so much better than I used to be. I look back and almost don't recognize the person I was. Being tired all the time was so exhausting and life-limiting. It feels so good to finally be enjoying my life in a career I am really passionate about and living my life to the full.

If I am being truthful with myself, I will always have to manage my energy. I notice that if I stray too far away from my new lifestyle – perhaps I have a bit too much sugar or pack in too many social plans – the sheer exhaustion can come back. If I have a long good stint, I can kid myself that it's OK to eat whatever I want, but the truth is, I can't. When this happens, the only way to describe it is I become lethargic, unproductive and need copious amounts of rest.

When I consciously manage my energy and am consistent, incorporating all the little changes into my daily life from this book, I thrive. There are days when I am not perfect, and that is OK. Sometimes I still like to live a little and indulge in some of my favourite foods that, truthfully, I know my gut doesn't love, but the pain and tiredness that ensue really aren't worth it.

I can imagine you now feeling so tired and wanting desperately to feel differently. It can be so hard to start. I have been there and I know how you feel. But I really hope that once you finish reading this book, you'll feel it's possible to change perhaps just one tiny thing and take a big step towards regaining your energy. It is about consistency, not perfection; self-compassion, not dieting or deprivation.

I just urge you not to ignore the signs your body is giving you as there can be serious health consequences for doing so. Being tired all the time is not normal and it's time for you to invest in yourself. You have the power to reverse your fatigue. Best of luck with your energy journey and please feel free to reach out if you need any support or advice.

5-MINUTE HACKS TO INCREASE ENERGY

- nutrient-dense snack, such as an apple and nut butter, + 3 minutes breathing
- 5-minute restorative shut-eye
- 15 squats + 3 minutes of stretching
- 5-minute walk in the fresh air
- 5 minutes of doing absolutely nothing
- one shot of fermented foods per day

Notes Page

To jot down thoughts, meal ideas, shopping lists or start your morning pages.

....

....

....

....

....

....

....

....

....

....

....

Notes Page

....

....

....

....

....

....

....

....

....

....

....

....

....

....

....

....

....

Glossary of Terms

Absorption = small intestine breaks down nutrients that are then absorbed into your bloodstream and carried to cells through your body.

Adrenal fatigue = adrenals are two glands that sit over your kidneys. Adrenal fatigue occurs when the adrenals have been overworked and can no longer secrete levels of cortisol that are adequate for optimal function.

Allergy = when your immune system reacts to a foreign substance — such as pollen or food that doesn't cause a reaction in most people. The immune system produces substances known as antibodies. When you have allergies, your immune system makes antibodies that identify a particular allergen as harmful, even though it isn't.

Amino acid = these are the molecules that all living things need to make protein. Nine of them are essential – histidine, isoleucine, leucine, lysine, methionine, phenylalanine, threonine, tryptophan, and valine which you have to get from the food you eat, the rest are conditional or non essential.

Anaemia = also known as low haemoglobin, is a condition where you lack enough healthy red blood cells to carry adequate oxygen to your body's tissues.

Antioxidant = a molecule that neutralizes free radicals in the body. Antioxidants donate an electron or take one away from the free radical to make it stable.

Anxiety = is your body's natural response to stress. It's a feeling of fear or apprehension about what's to come. It can be your body's way of telling you that something isn't quite right.

ADH – alcohol dehydrogenase = a class of zinc enzymes which is our primary defence against alcohol, a toxic molecule that compromises the function of our nervous system.

ADP – adenosine diphosphate = is an important organic compound in metabolism and is essential to the flow of energy in living cells.

ALDH – aldehyde dehydrogenase = primary enzymes involved in alcohol metabolism along with alcohol dehydrogenase.

ATP – adenosine triphosphate = energy-carrying molecule found in the cells of all living things. It consists of three components: a nitrogenous base (adenine), the sugar ribose, and the triphosphate.

Autoimmunity = when the immune system is dysregulated and makes a mistake, causing it to attack the body's own tissues or organs.

Bioavailability = refers to the proportion or fraction of a nutrient, consumed in the diet, that is absorbed and utilized by the body.

Biodiversity = is essential for the processes that support humans and all life on Earth. Without a wide range of animals, plants and microorganisms, we cannot have the healthy ecosystems that we rely on to provide us with the air we breathe and the food we eat.

Burnout = a state of physical or emotional exhaustion that also involves a sense of reduced accomplishment and loss of personal identity.

Carbohydrate = a type of macronutrient along with protein and fats that are the main source of energy for the body. They are the sugars, starches, and dietary fibre that occur in plant foods and dairy products.

Cell = the basic membrane-bound unit that contains the fundamental molecules of life and of which all living things are composed.

Circadian rhythm = Circadian rhythm is the name given to your body's 24-hour 'internal clock.' This internal clock controls your body's sleep–wake cycle.

Co-infection = is the simultaneous infection of a host by multiple pathogen species, for instance multi-parasite infection.

Chronotype = classification of when your genetic propensity is to sleep. It's determined by the PER3 gene.

CRP (c-reactive protein) = is a substance the liver produces in response to inflammation. A high level of CRP in the blood can be a marker of inflammation.

Cytokine = small and membrane-bound protein-based agents that modulate or alter the immune system response. They aid cell-to-cell communication in immune responses and stimulate the movement of cells towards sites of inflammation, infection and trauma.

Depression = is a mood disorder that causes a persistent feeling of sadness and loss of interest.

Digestion = the complex process of turning the food you eat into nutrients, which the body uses for energy, growth and cell repair needed to survive.

Dopamine = is one of several neurotransmitters strongly linked with mood and sensations of pleasure.

Dysbiosis = an 'imbalance' in the gut microbial community that is associated with disease.

Electron = is a negatively charged subatomic particle that together with protons and neutrons form an atom's nucleus.

Electron transport chain = releases the energy stored within the reduced hydrogen carriers in order to synthesise ATP. This is called *oxidative phosphorylation*, as the energy to synthesise ATP is derived from the oxidation of hydrogen carriers.

Epigenetics = is the study of how your behaviours and environment can cause changes that affect the way your genes work.

ESR (erythrocyte sedimentation rate) = is a blood test that checks for inflammation in your body.

Fat = the body uses fat as a fuel source, and fat is the major storage form of energy in the body. Fat also has many other important functions in the body, and a moderate amount is needed in the diet for good health. Fats in food come in several forms, including saturated, monounsaturated, and polyunsaturated.

Food intolerance = a food intolerance is when the body can't properly digest the food that is eaten, or that a particular food might irritate the digestive system.

Free radicals = are unstable atoms that can damage cells, causing illness and ageing.

Functional medicine = is a systems biology-based approach that focuses on identifying and addressing the root cause of disease.

GABA = a chemical made in the brain. As an inhibitory neurotransmitter, GABA reduces a nerve cell's ability to send and receive chemical messages throughout the central nervous system.

Genetics = studies how individual genes or groups of genes are involved in health and disease.

Glucose = a simple sugar with the molecular formula $C_6 H_{12} O_6$. Glucose is overall the most abundant monosaccharide, a subcategory of carbohydrates.

Glycine = one of the many amino acids your body needs to function properly. Glycine stimulates production of the 'feel good' hormone serotonin and serves as a key component of collagen, a protein that gives structure to bones, skin, muscles and connective tissues.

Gut microbiome = are the microorganisms, including bacteria, archaea, fungi, and viruses that live inside the digestive tracts.

Haem iron = a precursor to haemoglobin, which is necessary to bind oxygen in the bloodstream.

Haemoglobin = is a protein in your red blood cells. Your red blood cells carry oxygen throughout your body.

Hedonic adaptation = also known as the '*hedonic treadmill*' is a positive psychology theory that suggests people repeatedly return to their baseline level of happiness, regardless of what happens to them. An example being winning the lottery.

Homeostatic sleep drive = also known as sleep pressure, is a biological process part of the two-process model controlling sleep.

Hyperthyroidism = (overactive thyroid) happens when the thyroid gland makes too much thyroid hormone.

Hypothroidism = (underactive thyroid) is a condition in which your thyroid gland doesn't produce enough of certain crucial hormones.

Inflammation = occurs when your immune system sends out cells to fight bacteria or heal an injury. Chronic inflammation can cause health problems.

Insulin = is a hormone made in your pancreas. It helps your body use glucose (sugar) for energy.

Insulin resistance = is when cells in your muscles, fat, and liver don't respond well to insulin and can't use glucose from your blood for energy.

Intuitive eating = is about trusting your inner body wisdom to make choices around food that feel good in your body, without judgment and without influence from diet culture.

Macronutrient = are the nutrients we need in larger quantities that provide us with energy: in other words, fat, protein and carbohydrate.

Malabsorption = occurs when people are unable to absorb nutrients from their diets, such as carbohydrates, fats, minerals, proteins.

Melatonin = is a hormone that your brain produces in response to darkness. It helps with the timing of your circadian rhythms (24-hour internal clock) and with sleep. Being exposed to light at night can block melatonin production.

Metabolic dysfunction = occurs when the metabolism process fails and causes the body to have either too much or too little of the essential substances needed to stay healthy. Metabolic syndrome is the medical term for a combination of diabetes, high blood pressure (hypertension) and obesity.

Micronutrient = are mostly vitamins and minerals, and are equally important but consumed in very small amounts.

Mitochondria = are organelles in the cell and often referred to as the powerhouses of the cell. They help turn the energy we take from food into energy that the cell can use.

Nutrient density = is the ratio of beneficial ingredients to the food's energy content for the amount that is commonly consumed.

Oestrogen = one of the main female sex hormones. It is needed for puberty, the menstrual cycle, pregnancy, bone strength and other functions of the body. Oestrogen levels vary throughout the menstrual cycle and fall after menopause.

Organelle = is a subcellular structure that has one or more specific jobs to perform in the cell, much like an organ does in the body.

Organism = an organism is any organic, living system that functions as an individual entity. All organisms are composed of cells.

Orthorexic = an unhealthy obsession with eating 'pure' food. Food considered 'pure' or 'impure' can vary from person to person.

Oxalates = are a type of compound found naturally in a variety of foods, including certain types of fruits, vegetables, beans, nuts, and grains.

Oxidation = is the loss of electrons during a reaction by a molecule, atom or ion.

Oxidative stress = is an imbalance between free radicals and antioxidants in your body.

Non-haem iron = is found in plant foods like whole grains, nuts, seeds, legumes and leafy greens.

Nudge theory = is a branch of behavioural economics and seeks to understand how people think, make decisions, and behave.

Nutrigenomics = is a science studying the relationship between human genome, human nutrition and health.

Pica = is an eating disorder in which people compulsively eat one or more nonfood items, such as ice, clay, paper, ash or dirt.

Positive psychology = seeks to understand the factors that allow individuals, communities and societies to flourish.

Progesterone = is a hormone that's vital for menstruation, pregnancy, and sperm production.

Protein = is a macronutrient that plays many critical roles in the body. They do most of the work in cells and are required for the structure, function, and regulation of the body's tissues and organs.

RDA – recommended daily allowance = average daily level of intake sufficient to meet the nutrient requirements of nearly all (97–98%) healthy individuals.

REM – rapid eye movement = during sleep, the brain moves through four different stages. One of these stages is rapid eye movement (REM) sleep. During this phase, the eyes move rapidly in various directions.

Respiration = is the chemical process by which organic compounds release energy.

ROS – radical oxygen species = is a type of unstable molecule that contains oxygen and easily reacts with other molecules in a cell. A build-up of reactive oxygen species in cells may cause damage to DNA, RNA, and proteins, and may cause cell death. Reactive oxygen species are free radicals.

SAD – seasonal affective disorder = this type of depression is related to changes in seasons and begins and ends at about the same times every year.

Set point theory = states that the human body tries to maintain its weight within a preferred range.

Serotonin = is a hormone and neurotransmitter, and is sometimes known as the happy chemical. It appears to play a role in regulating mood.

TEF – thermic effect of food = is the amount of energy it takes for your body to digest, absorb, and metabolize the food you eat.

Testosterone = is the male sex hormone that is made in the testicles. Testosterone hormone levels are important to normal male sexual development and functions.

Toxins = are substances created by plants and animals that are poisonous (toxic) to humans.

Tryptophan = is an amino acid needed for normal growth in infants and for the production and maintenance of the body's proteins, muscles, enzymes and neurotransmitters.

Virus = is an infectious agent of small size and simple composition that can multiply only in living cells of animals, plants or bacteria.

Resources Directory

Back when I was feeling really unwell with burnout, I remember not knowing where to turn and feeling so helpless. Here is a list of useful resources, products, apps and websites to support you on your journey.

Find a reputable nutritionist

The email for my practice is hello@nocohealth.co.uk. If you get really stuck, I am happy to try and point you in the right direction. Join my newsletter for my energy tips every week @ www.nocohealth.co.uk

I also have a course that will guide you through your Five Step plan and can support you virtually on your journey here: www.nocohealth.co.uk/pages/fixyourfatigue

You can also follow us on Instagram @karina_antram.

When you are choosing who to work with, make sure:

- They offer a call first without charge. You need to ensure they are the right person to support you or they should be referring you to someone else.
- You understand their credentials, that they are accredited with their industry bodies and you feel confident that they can add value to your case.

Questions to ask any practitioner you may want to work with:

- What accredited bodies are you a member of?
- What qualifications do you have?
- What are your specialisms?
- Can you talk me through what your consultation/ programme entails?
- What are your fees? (Understand the full costs upfront.)
- Would you suggest any testing? If so, where do you get your tests from and how much are they? (Testing can be really expensive, so do be careful before agreeing to any tests.) You may want to hold off on testing if the symptom can be alleviated through diet and lifestyle interventions first.

Make a doctor's appointment

Check the red flag list on pages 89–90 in this book and mention any of them to your doctor. Remember to include all your symptoms.

Emergency doctor numbers

UK: 111
Germany: 116117
Spain: 1003
France: 15 or 112
US: 911
Canada: 811
Australia: 1800 022 222
South Africa: 10111 or 10177

BANT – British Association for Nutrition and Lifestyle Medicine (UK governing body)
https://practitioner-search.bant.org.uk

IFM – The Institute for Functional Medicine (global body)
https://www.ifm.org/find-a-practitioner

Student nutrition clinics

If your budget doesn't allow you to see a practitioner, there are many student clinics that offer discounted nutritionist rates starting from £25.

UK

The College of Naturopathic Medicine (London, Belfast, Birmingham, Brighton, Bristol, Edinburgh, Manchester)

These are student clinics and they are practising their craft, so the service will differ, but they are supervised by a qualified practitioner.

https://www.naturopathy-uk.com/resources/
student-clinics/

The Institute of Optimum Nutrition
https://www.ion.ac.uk/pages/category/
optimum-nutrition-clinic

Blood tests
If you want to check your bloods at home:

Thriva
https://thriva.co

Medichecks
https://medichecks.com

Functional tests to be done through a qualified practitioner:

Nordic Labs
http://nordiclabs.com

Genova Diagnostics
https://www.gdx.net/uk/

Invivo
https://invivohealthcare.com

Regenerus
https://regeneruslabs.com

Gut tests

Zoe
https://joinzoe.com/gut-test-v2

Food allergy testing

York
https://www.yorktest.com

STEP 1: FUEL YOUR BODY

Local honey or manuka brands

UK
https://localfoodbritain.com/london/food/honey/
https://www.localhoneyfinder.org

Comvita
https://www.comvita.co.uk

Allotments

You can apply for a plot of land via your council
https://www.gov.uk/apply-allotment

Water filters

Fresh Water Filter
https://www.freshwaterfilter.com

Healthy House
https://healthy-house.co.uk

Coffee brands

Coffee: Exhale Coffee
https://exhalecoffee.com

Dandelion: Aquasol
https://aquasol.co.uk

Mushroom: London Nootropics
https://londonnootropics.com

Merryhill Mushrooms
https://www.merryhill-mushrooms.co.uk

Teas

Pukka
https://www.pukkaherbs.com

Alcohol free

Seedlip
https://www.seedlipdrinks.com

Gin
Clean Co
https://clean.co

Wine
Wild Idol
https://wildidol.com

Seaweed and other sea vegetables

Clearspring
https://www.clearspring.co.uk/collections/
organic-wild-harvested-sea-vegetables

STEP 2: SUPPORT YOUR GUT

You can make the following yourself at home, but if you are
time-poor:

Yoghurt

Choose full-fat natural yoghurt, never low-fat and ideally not flavoured yoghurts.

Sauerkraut

Profusion Organic
https://www.profusionorganic.co.uk/products/profusion-organic-fresh-sauerkraut/

Biona
https://biona.co.uk/product/biona-organic-sauerkraut

Kombucha

Momo
https://momo-kombucha.com

GTS Living
https://gtslivingfoods.com

Kefir

Chuckling Goat
https://www.chucklinggoat.co.uk

The Collective Dairy
https://www.thecollectivedairy.com

Non-toxic cleaning products

Ecover
https://www.ecoverdirect.com

Method
https://www.methodshop.co.uk

Honest
https://www.honest.com

We Are Spruce
https://www.wearespruce.co

Cheeky Panda
https://uk.cheekypanda.com

Smol
https://smolproducts.com

Bio-D
https://biod.co.uk

Skin and bodycare brands

Tropic
https://tropicskincare.com

Green People
https://www.greenpeople.co.uk

The Organic Pharmacy
https://www.theorganicpharmacy.com

Tarte Cosmetics
https://tartecosmetics.com/EU/en_GB/home/

Ranavat
https://www.ranavat.com

Gaia
https://www.gaiaskincare.com

Monks
https://monks.world

Alumier
https://www.alumiermd.co.uk

Blue Alchemy
https://www.perfectbluealchemy.com

Makeup

Saie
https://saiehello.com

Ilia

https://iliabeauty.com

Jane Iredale

https://janeiredale.com

Comfort Zone

https://world.comfortzoneskin.com

STEP 3: SUPERCHARGE YOUR SLEEP AND EXERCISE

Meditation apps

Headspace

https://www.headspace.com

Calm

https://www.calm.com

Online yoga

Yoga with Adriene

https://www.youtube.com/user/yogawithadriene/
videos?app=desktop

Magnesium salts

West Lab

https://westlabsalts.co.uk

Better You
https://betteryou.com/products/magnesium-flakes

STEP 4: ENERGIZE WITH SUPPLEMENTS

As we have learnt, there are lots of poor-quality supplements out there. Many reputable supplement companies have their own clinical teams that you can speak to if you need any product advice.

Natural Dispensary
https://naturaldispensary.co.uk (only possible via a practitioner)

Revital
https://www.revital.co.uk

Naturisimo
https://www.naturisimo.com

France
Nutrixeal
nutrixeal.fr

UNAE
unae.fr

Sunday Natural
https://sunday.fr/

Energetic Natura
energeticanatura.com

Bionutrics
https://www.bionutrics.fr/

US
Pure Encapsulations
https://www.pureencapsulations.com

Thorne
https://www.thorne.com

Sweden
Simris
https://www.simris.com

Reputable supplement brands

UK
£
Optibac https://www.optibacprobiotics.com
Lambert's https://www.lambertshealthcare.co.uk
Better You https://betteryou.com
Solgar https://solgar.co.uk
Culturelle https://www.culturelle.com

££

BioCare https://www.biocare.co.uk
Nature's Aid https://www.naturesaid.co.uk
Bionutri https://www.bionutri.co.uk
Wild Nutrition https://www.wildnutrition.com
Nutri Advanced https://www.nutriadvanced.co.uk
Cytoplan https://www.cytoplan.co.uk

£££

Thorne https://www.thorne.com
Activated Probiotics https://activatedprobiotics.com.au
Pure Encapsulations https://www.pureencapsulations.com

Sign up to their newsletters and look out for their sales as this can save you a lot of money.

STEP 5: HARNESS THE POWER OF YOUR BRAIN

Find a therapist

If you need to talk to someone, Mind is a good place to start.
https://www.mind.org.uk/information-support/drugs-and-treatments/talking-therapy-and-counselling/how-to-find-a-therapist/

Personality test (*understanding yourself better*)

https://www.16personalities.com/free-personality-test
https://www.viacharacter.org/survey/account/Register

How to find a coach

If you have read the first half of the book and you think your tiredness may be due to your career or life choices, you may want to see a coach.

You can find a qualified coach through the **International Coaching Federation**:

https://coachingfederation.org

SHOPPING LIST OF BASIC INGREDIENTS TO FILL YOUR STORE CUPBOARD AND GET YOU STARTED

Fridge
Eggs
Full-fat butter

Dairy/non-dairy
Greek or coconut yoghurt
Milk or plant-based milk, such as cashew, hazelnut, almond, coconut

Fruit
Avocados
Berries, apples, bananas
Frozen berries are fine or opt for what fruit is in season – eat whatever else you love, but mix it up

Vegetables
Green leafy vegetables, such as spinach, kale, spring greens, Swiss chard – eat whatever else you love but mix it up
Sweet or white potatoes

Sweets

Dark chocolate

Honey

Maple syrup

Store cupboard

Apple cider vinegar

Beans – cannellini beans (tinned), kidney beans (tinned), butter beans (tinned), black-eyed beans (tinned)

Chickpeas (tinned)

Coconut oil, olive oil and ghee

Lentils

Nut butter

Nuts (if no allergy), such as almonds, cashews, hazelnuts, walnuts and Brazil nuts

Passata

Pasta – try a different range – wholemeal, white, spelt, brown rice, red lentil, chickpea and spinach

Porridge oats

Quinoa

Rice – try a different range – brown, white, basmati, red and black

Rye bread or sourdough

Salt and pepper

Seeds – mix omega-rich seeds, such as pumpkin, chia, sunflower and flaxseed

Spices – such as cumin seeds, rosemary, basil, thyme, smoked paprika, garlic powder, oregano, cinnamon, turmeric and ginger

Stock cubes

Tinned chopped tomatoes

Tinned coconut milk

Tinned tuna

Tomato paste

Freezer

Acai, for smoothies and smoothie bowls

Bananas

Berries

Broad beans

Green beans

Kale

Peas

Spinach

Sweetcorn

Meal ideas from the previous ingredients list

Breakfast: Avocado and feta on toast; porridge with berries and nut butter; scrambled eggs on toast with seeds; no-flour banana pancakes with berries, seeds and Greek yoghurt

Lunch: Dhal and rice with broccoli; vegetarian bolognese with pasta; sweetcorn fritters; avocado, feta and pea smash; smoked sesame salmon poke bowl; smoky baked beans on sweet potato or rye toast

Dinner: Baked fish with oil and lemon, green beans, crushed new buttered potatoes; tuna steak, noodles and tangy orange dressing; kimchi mince buddha bowl; chicken nasi goreng; tofu stir-fry with pak choi

Snack ideas: Dark chocolate (min. 70%) dipped strawberries covered in crushed hazelnuts; banana, avocado and date smoothie; rye toast and hummus with seeds; apple with nut butter; Greek yoghurt; passion fruit/pomegranate seeds with nuts/seeds

Deprivation this is not! All these meals are also perfect for children if they are not allergic to any of the ingredients. This will save you time making extra meals for adults and children and many of them are suitable for batch cooking.

If you need some extra help to get you started, these are some meal delivery companies

Mindful Chef https://www.mindfulchef.com
Hello Fresh https://www.hellofresh.co.uk

Organic food boxes
Abel & Cole https://www.abelandcole.co.uk
Riverford https://www.riverford.co.uk
Oddbox (not organic for wonky fruit and vegetables)
  https://www.oddbox.co.uk
Eversfield https://eversfieldorganic.co.uk

Farmers' markets
London
https://www.lfm.org.uk

UK
https://saturdayandsunday.co.uk/
weekend-farmers-market-directory/

Recommended further reading
Life Time by Russell Foster
Energize by Simon Alexander Ong
Atomic Habits by James Clear
The High 5 Habit by Mel Robbins

RECAP

- Be honest with your doctor about *all* your symptoms.
- There is always a way forward – contact us @noco health if you feel stuck.
- Make sure you have a free call first before enlisting any practitioner.
- Check their credentials and make sure they are accredited to a relevant body.

References

Chapter 1: Why Am I So Tired?

Micklewright, D., St Clair Gibson, A., Gladwell, V. & Al Salman, A. (2017). Development and Validity of the Rating-of-Fatigue Scale. *Sports Medicine (Auckland, N.Z.)*, 47(11), 2375–93. https://doi.org/10.1007/s40279-017-0711-5

Chapter 2: Who Stole My Energy?

Aron, Elaine, *The Highly Sensitive Person: How to Thrive When the World Overwhelms You* (Thorsons, 1999)

Deary, V., Hagenaars S.P., Harris, S.E., et al. (2018). Genetic Contributions to Self-reported Tiredness [published correction appears in *Mol Psychiatry*, Mar; 23 (3):789–90]. *Mol Psychiatry*. 2018;23(3):609–20. doi:10.1038/mp.2017.5

Greenberg, Donna B. (2002). Clinical Dimensions of Fatigue. *Primary Care Companion to the Journal of Clinical Psychiatry* vol. 4,3: 90–93. doi:10.4088/pcc.v04n0301

Hyder, F., Rothman, D. L., & Bennett, M. R. (2013). Cortical Energy Demands of Signalling and Non-signalling Components in the Brain

References

Are Conserved Across Mammalian Species and Activity Levels. *Proc. Natl. Acad. Sci. USA* 110, 3549–54. doi: 10.1073/pnas.1214912110

Jiang, P., & Turek, F. W. (2018). The Endogenous Circadian Clock Programs Animals to Eat at Certain Times of the 24-hour Day: What If We Ignore the Clock? *Physiology & Behaviour, 193*(Pt B), 211–17. https://doi.org/10.1016/j.physbeh.2018.04.017

Kanerva, N., Kronholm, E., Partonen, T., Ovaskainen, M. L., Kaartinen, N. E., Konttinen, H., Broms, U., & Männistö, S. (2012). Tendency Toward Eveningness Is Associated with Unhealthy Dietary Habits. *Chronobiology International, 29*(7), 920–27. https://doi.org/10.3109/07420528.2012.699128

Lee, I. M., Shiroma, E. J., Kamada, M., Bassett, D. R., Matthews, C. E., & Buring, J. E. (2019). Association of Step Volume and Intensity with All-Cause Mortality in Older Women. *JAMA Internal Medicine, 179*(8), 1105–12. https://doi.org/10.1001/jamainternmed.2019.0899

Lewina O. Lee, PhD, Francine Grodstein, ScD, Claudia Trudel-Fitzgerald, PhD, Peter James, ScD, Sakurako S. Okuzono, MPH, Hayami K. Koga, MD, Joel Schwartz, PhD, Avron Spiro, III, PhD, Daniel K. Mroczek, PhD, Laura D. Kubzansky, PhD. (2022). Optimism, Daily Stressors, and Emotional Well-Being Over Two Decades in a Cohort of Ageing Men. *The Journals of Gerontology: Series B*, 2022; gbac025, https://doi.org/10.1093/geronb/gbac025

Martínez Steele, E., Baraldi, L.G., Louzada, M.L.D.C., et al. (2016). Ultra-Processed Foods and Added Sugars in the US Diet: Evidence from a Nationally Representative Cross-sectional Study. *BMJ Open* 2016; **6:**e 009892. doi: 10.1136/bmjopen-2015-009892

Maté, Gabor, *When the Body Says No: Understanding the Stress-Disease Connection* (John Wiley & Sons, 2003)

Maukonen, M., Kanerva, N., Pärtonen, T., Kronholm, E., Konttinen, H., Wennman, H. & Männistö S. (2016). The Associations between Chronotype, a Healthy Diet and Obesity. *Chronobiology International*, 33:8, 972–81. doi: 10.1080/07420528.2016.1183022

Mohebi, A., Pettibone, J. R., Hamid, A. A. et al. (2019). Dissociable Dopamine Dynamics for Learning and Motivation. *Nature* 570, 65–70. https://doi.org/10.1038/s41586-019-1235-y

Rauber, F., Louzada, M.L.D.C., Martinez Steele, E., et al. (2019). Ultra-processed Foods and Excessive Free Sugar Intake in the UK: a Nationally Representative Cross-sectional Study. *BMJ Open* 2019; 9:e 027546. doi: 10.1136/bmjopen-2018-027546

Spreng, R.N., Dimas, E., Mwilambwe-Tshilobo, L. et al. (2020). The Default Network of the Human Brain Is Associated with Perceived Social Isolation. *Nat Commun* 11, 6393. https://doi.org/10.1038/s41467-020-20039-w

Oishi, Y., Xu, Q., Wang, L., Zhang, B.-J., Takahashi, K., Takata, Y., Luo, Y.-J., Cherasse, Y., Schiffmann, S. N., de Kerchove d'Exaerde, A., Urade, Y., Qu, W. M., Huang, Z. L., Lazarus, M. (2017). Slow-wave Sleep Is Controlled by a Subset of Nucleus Accumbens Core Neurons in Mice. *Nature Communications*, 8 (1). doi: 10.1038/s41467-017-00781-4

Chapter 3: How Can I Mend My Broken Mitochondria?

https://drmyhill.co.uk/wiki/d-ribose

Flockhart, M., Nilsson, L. C., Tais, S., Ekblom, B., Apró, W. & Larsen, F. J. (2021). Excessive exercise training causes mitochondrial functional impairment and decreases glucose tolerance in healthy volunteers. *Cell metabolism*, *33*(5), 957–70.e6. https://doi.org/10.1016/j.cmet.2021.02.017

Segerstrom, S. C. (2007). Stress, Energy, and Immunity: An Ecological View. *Current Directions in Psychological Science, 16*(6), 326–30. https://doi.org/10.1111/j.1467-8721.2007.00522.x

van der Kolk, B., Saari, S., Lovric, A., Arif, M., Alvarez, M., Ko, A., Miao, Z., Sahebekhtiari, N., Muniandy, M., Heinonen, S., Oghabian, A., Jokinen, R., Jukarainen, S., Hakkarainen, A., Lundbom, J., Kuula, J., Groop, P.-H., Tukiainen, T., Lundbom, N., Rissanen, A., Kaprio, J., Williams, E., Zamboni, N., Mardinoglu, A., Pajukanta, P., Pietiläinen, K. H. (2021). Molecular Pathways behind Acquired Obesity: Adipose Tissue and Skeletal Muscle Multi Omics in Monozygotic Twin Pairs Discordant for BMI. *Cell Reports Medicine*, 2021. doi: 10.1016/j.xcrm.2021.100226

Chapter 4: What Else Could Be Wrong?

https://acaai.org/allergies/allergies-101/facts-stats/

https://www.veroval.info/-/media/diagnostics/files/knowledge/eaaci_advocacy_manifesto.pdf

Bikman, Benjamin, PhD, *Why We Get Sick* (BenBella Books, 2020)

Lee, J. S., Kim, H. G., Lee, D. S. & Son, C. G. (2018). Oxidative Stress is a Convincing Contributor to Idiopathic Chronic Fatigue. *Scientific Reports*, 8(1), 12890. https://doi.org/10.1038/s41598-018-31270-3

Munusamy, S. & MacMillan-Crow, L. A. (2009). Mitochondrial Superoxide Plays a Crucial Role in the Development of Mitochondrial Dysfunction during High Glucose Exposure in Rat Renal Proximal Tubular Cells. *Free. Radic. Biol. Med.* 46, 1149–57

References

Tirichen, H., Yaigoub, H., Xu, W., Wu, C., Li, R. & Li, Y. (2021). Mitochondrial Reactive Oxygen Species and Their Contribution in Chronic Kidney Disease Progression Through Oxidative Stress. *Frontiers in Physiology*, 12, 627837. https://doi.org/10.3389/fphys.2021.627837

Wood, E., Hall, K. H. & Tate, W. (2021). Role of Mitochondria, Oxidative Stress and the Response to Antioxidants in Myalgic Encephalomyelitis/Chronic Fatigue Syndrome: a Possible Approach to SARS-CoV-2 'Long-haulers'? *Chronic Diseases and Translational Medicine*, 7(1), 14–26. https://doi.org/10.1016/j.cdtm.2020.11.002

Zhao, N., Liu, C. C., Van Ingelgom, A. J., Martens, Y. A., Linares, C., Knight, J. A., Painter, M. M., Sullivan, P. M. & Bu, G. (2017). Apolipoprotein E4 Impairs Neuronal Insulin Signaling by Trapping Insulin Receptor in the Endosomes. *Neuron*, 96(1), 115–29.e5. https://doi.org/10.1016/j.neuron.2017.09.003

Chapter 5: Why Don't Doctors Have All the Answers?

Anand, P., Kunnumakkara, A. B., Sundaram, C., Harikumar, K. B., Tharakan, S. T., Lai, O. S., Sung, B. & Aggarwal, B. B. (2008). Cancer Is a Preventable Disease That Requires Major Lifestyle Changes. *Pharmaceutical Research*, 25(9), 2097–116. https://doi.org/10.1007/s11095-008-9661-9

Gaufin, T., Tobin, N.H., Aldrovandi, G.M. (2018). The Importance of the Microbiome in Paediatrics and Paediatric Infectious Diseases. *Curr Opin Pediatr*, 30(1):117–24. doi:1097/MOP.0000000000000576

Jackson, M. A., Verdi, S., Maxan, M. E., Shin, C. M., Zierer, J., Bowyer, R., Martin, T., Williams, F., Menni, C., Bell, J. T., Spector,

T. D. & Steves, C. J. (2018). Gut Microbiota Associations with Common Diseases and Prescription Medications in a Population-based Cohort. *Nature Communications*, 9(1), 2655. https://doi.org/10.1038/s41467-018-05184-7

Stiemsma, L.T., Michels, K.B. (2018). The Role of the Microbiome in the Developmental Origins of Health and Disease. *Pediatrics*; 141(4):e20172437. doi:1542/peds.2017-2437

Step 1: Fuel Your Body

Debbeler, L.J., Gamp, M., Blumenschein, M., Keim, D., Renner, B. (2018). Polarised but Illusory Beliefs about Tap and Bottled Water: a Product- and Consumer-oriented Survey and Blind Tasting Experiment. *Sci Total Environ*, 2018; 643:1400–10. doi:10.1016/j.scitotenv.2018.06.190

Freitas D, Boué F, Benallaoua M, Airinei G, Benamouzig R, Le Feunteun S. Lemon juice, but not tea, reduces the glycemic response to bread in healthy volunteers: a randomized crossover trial. Eur J Nutr. 2021 Feb;60(1):113-122. doi: 10.1007/s00394-020-02228-x. Epub 2020 Mar 23. PMID: 32201919.

González, S., Salazar, N., Ruiz-Saavedra, S., Gómez-Martín, M., de Los Reyes-Gavilán, C. G., & Gueimonde, M. (2020). Long-Term Coffee Consumption is Associated with Fecal Microbial Composition in Humans. *Nutrients*, 12(5), 1287. https://doi.org/10.3390/nu12051287

https://www.sciencedaily.com/releases/2021/08/210803175250.htm

Gordon, E. L., Ariel-Donges, A. H., Bauman, V., & Merlo, L. J. (2018). What Is the Evidence for 'Food Addiction?' A Systematic Review. *Nutrients*, 10(4), 477. https://doi.org/10.3390/nu10040477

Robertson, T. M., Clifford, M. N., Penson, S., Williams, P. & Robertson, M. D. (2018). Postprandial Glycaemic and Lipaemic Responses to Chronic Coffee Consumption May Be Modulated by CYP1A2 polymorphisms. *The British Journal of Nutrition*, *119*(7), 792–800. https://doi.org/10.1017/S0007114518000260

Step 2: Support Your Gut

Mayer, A. B., Trenchard, L. & Rayns, F. (2022). Historical Changes in the Mineral Content of Fruit and Vegetables in the UK from 1940 to 2019: a Concern for Human Nutrition and Agriculture. *International Journal of Food Sciences and Nutrition*, *73*(3), 315–26. https://doi.org/10.1080/09637486.2021.1981831

Step 3: Supercharge Your Sleep and Exercise

https://www.cdc.gov/niosh/work-hour-training-for-nurses/longhours/mod2/11.html

https://www.sleepfoundation.org/stages-of-sleep

https://www.cdc.gov/niosh/work-hour-training-for-nurses/longhours/mod2/11.html

Harrison, Y. & Horn, J.A. 'High sleep ability without sleepiness'. The ability to fall asleep rapidly without other signs of sleepiness. *Neurophysiol Clin.* 1996; 26(1):15–20. doi:10.1016/0987-7053(96)81530-9

Saner, N. J., Lee, M. J., Kuang, J., Pitchford, N. W., Roach, G. D., Garnham, A., Genders, A. J., Stokes, T., Schroder, E. A., Huo, Z., Esser, K. A., Phillips, S. M., Bishop, D. J. & Bartlett, J. D. (2021). Exercise Mitigates Sleep-loss-induced Changes in Glucose Tolerance, Mitochondrial Function, Sarcoplasmic Protein Synthesis, and Diurnal

Rhythms. *Molecular Metabolism*, 43, 101110. https://doi.org/10.1016/j.molmet.2020.101110

St-Onge, M. P., Mikic, A. & Pietrolungo, C. E. (2016). Effects of Diet on Sleep Quality. *Advances in Nutrition (Bethesda, Md.)*, 7(5), 938–49. https://doi.org/10.3945/an.116.012336

Step 4: Energize with Supplements

Candelario, M., Cuellar, E., Reyes-Ruiz, J.M. et al. (2015). Direct Evidence for GABAergic Activity of Withania Somnifera on Mammalian Ionotropic GABAA and GABAρ Receptors. *J Ethnopharmacol*; 171:264–72. doi:10.1016/j.jep.2015.05.058

Darmadi-Blackberry, I., Wahlqvist, M. L., Kouris-Blazos, A., Steen, B., Lukito, W., Horie, Y. & Horie, K. (2004). Legumes: the Most Important Dietary Predictor of Survival in Older People of Different Ethnicities. *Asia Pacific Journal of Clinical Nutrition*, 13(2), 217–20

Flanagan, J. L., Simmons, P. A., Vehige, J., Willcox, M. D. & Garrett, Q. (2010). Role of Carnitine in Disease. *Nutrition & Metabolism*, 7, 30. https://doi.org/10.1186/1743-7075-7-30

Hozayen, W. G., Mahmoud, A. M., Soliman, H. A. & Mostafa, S. R. (2016). Spirulina Versicolor Improves Insulin Sensitivity and Attenuates Hyperglycemia-mediated Oxidative Stress in Fructose-fed Rats. *Journal of Intercultural Ethnopharmacology*, 5(1), 57–64. https://doi.org/10.5455/jice.20151230055930

Wolfe, K. L., Kang, X., He, X., Dong, M., Zhang, Q. & Liu, R. H. (2008). *Journal of Agricultural and Food Chemistry* 56 (18), 8418–26. doi: 10.1021/jf801381y

Sanz-Milone, V., Yoshinori, P., & Maculano Esteves, A. (2021). Sleep quality of professional e-Sports athletes (Counter Strike: Global Offensive). International Journal of Esports, 1(1). Retrieved from https://www.ijesports.org/article/45/html

Wolfe, D., *Superfoods: The Food and Medicine of the Future* (California: North Atlantic Books, 2009) 10–49

Step 5: Harness the Power of Your Brain

Cameron, Julia, *The Artist's Way* (Souvenir Press, 2020)

Martin, K., Meeusen, R., Thompson, K.G. et al. (2018). Mental Fatigue Impairs Endurance Performance: a Physiological Explanation. *Sports Med* 48, 2041–51. https://doi.org/10.1007/s40279-018-0946-9

Tseng, J. & Poppenk, J. (2020). Brain Meta-state Transitions Demarcate Thoughts across Task Contexts Exposing the Mental Noise of Trait Neuroticism. *Nat Commun* 11, 3480. https://doi.org/10.1038/s41467-020-17255-9

Wieth, M. & Zacks, R. (2011). Time of Day Effects on Problem Solving: When the Non-optimal Is Optimal. *Thinking and Reasoning, 17* (4), 387–401. doi: 10.1080/13546783.2011.625663

Biography

Photo © Jodi Johnston

Karina Antram (BSc (hons), DIP-NT) is a registered nutritionist and graduate of the renowned College of Naturopathic Medicine and an executive coach.

Karina is hugely passionate about health and wellbeing after her own health struggles led her to seek out naturopathic practices. After being diagnosed with IBS, Chronic Fatigue Syndrome and Lyme disease, Karina tried out a multitude of tests, diets, health practices, different foods and herbs to try to combat her debilitating symptoms, which, at times, led her to being hospitalized. Karina is now recovered, having made numerous changes to her diet and lifestyle, but is fully aware that consistency and continuity are key.

Prior to becoming a Nutritionist, Karina spent 15 years working as an HR leader for organizations such as The Boston Consulting Group and Deloitte. She studied Biomedicine at The Institute of Optimum Nutrition and is currently a member of three governing bodies in the industry: BANT, ANP and CNHC. She is also a member of the Institute of Functional Medicine based in the US and a management graduate from Leeds University Business School. Follow Karina @karina_antram

Acknowledgements

I feel lucky to have had many positive influences in my life, who have actively contributed to getting to this point today.

To my mum, the secret poet, for giving me a love of reading and writing through the countless hours you spent with us as children. It is only now that I am a mother, I appreciate how selfless you were. To my dad for believing in me, actively encouraging my crazy business ideas and being willing to listen and support every single one of them. You never said I was mad, just go for it. Always. Watching you build your business from nothing has been very inspiring.

My partner Mark, for all the conversations, hours spent helping with childcare, making breakfast in bed so I could write first thing in the morning and listening to my ideas even after a long day at work. None of this would have been possible without your support. Thank you. My incredible son Billy for being an amazing, easy baby, which meant I had time during his naps to write early in the morning and in the evenings. I don't think this book would have been written without becoming a mother to you. All this is for you. My sister Lucy Gardner and brother-in-law James Gardner for all your valued input. Your advice was always spot on and appreciated. My grandparents Ann Antram and John Antram for teaching me to appreciate good quality food and nutrition from a very young age.

Ione Walder at Penguin Random House for taking a risk on a complete unknown without a social media platform. It really did change my life and meant the world. Daniel Hurst and Agatha Russell for all the editing, feedback and hard work to make this book what it is. Beatrix McIntyre and Kay Halsey for their copyediting. Courtney Barclay and Olivia Thomas for marketing and PR support. Sophie Bradshaw for being such a fantastic editor to work with. The team at my literary agent Graham Maw Christie, Jane Graham Maw and Jen Christie, for all the input, support and advice, and Maddy Belton for being a great first literary agent.

To my wonderful beta readers – Charlie Girling, Jodi Johnston, Benjamin Bell, Lucy Mullins, Lindsey Predergast, Katherine Horstmann and Nicola Peplow. My fantastic coach Jess Dooley for helping to keep the momentum going and being such an inspirational person to work with.

Beverly Glick for being so kind and taking time during the festive holiday season to help me get the book polished. I am eternally grateful.

Sue Richardson and the Right Book Buddies – Clare Norman, Mary Fenwick, Dave Plunkett, Dr Heather Cairns Lee, Mark Faithfull, Rachel Bentley, Paul Harris, Mary Andrews, Morton Patterson and Chantal Cornelius for all the wonderful words of wisdom and coaching.

Acknowledgements

The College of Naturopathic Medicine and Hermann Keppler. My supervisor Katarina Cepinova. My lecturers, Simon Bradley, Juliana Bernardes, Dr Jodi Cahill, Rhian Jones, Adam Greer, Keris Marsden, Kathy Pasch, Holly Taylor, Belle Amatt, Dr Marc Bubbs and Dr Sarah Myhill. Elizabeth Haylett Clarke and the Society of Authors. The London Writers Salon, Matt and Parul and Jamie Vickery.

He just wanted a decent book to read ...

Not too much to ask, is it? It was in 1935 when Allen Lane, Managing Director of Bodley Head Publishers, stood on a platform at Exeter railway station looking for something good to read on his journey back to London. His choice was limited to popular magazines and poor-quality paperbacks – the same choice faced every day by the vast majority of readers, few of whom could afford hardbacks. Lane's disappointment and subsequent anger at the range of books generally available led him to found a company – and change the world.

'We believed in the existence in this country of a vast reading public for intelligent books at a low price, and staked everything on it'
Sir Allen Lane, 1902–1970, founder of Penguin Books

The quality paperback had arrived – and not just in bookshops. Lane was adamant that his Penguins should appear in chain stores and tobacconists, and should cost no more than a packet of cigarettes.

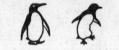

Reading habits (and cigarette prices) have changed since 1935, but Penguin still believes in publishing the best books for everybody to enjoy. We still believe that good design costs no more than bad design, and we still believe that quality books published passionately and responsibly make the world a better place.

So wherever you see the little bird – whether it's on a piece of prize-winning literary fiction or a celebrity autobiography, political tour de force or historical masterpiece, a serial-killer thriller, reference book, world classic or a piece of pure escapism – you can bet that it represents the very best that the genre has to offer.

Whatever you like to read – trust Penguin.